HYPNOTHERAPY

A SURVEY OF THE LITERATURE

HYPNOTHERAPY

A SURVEY OF THE LITERATURE

By MARGARET BRENMAN, PH. D.
Director of the Division of Psychology
The Menninger Foundation
Professor of Psychology
The Menninger Foundation Center
of the Department of Psychology
University of Kansas

&

MERTON M. GILL, M. D.
Associate Psychiatrist
Assistant Director, Department of Research
The Menninger Foundation

*With Appended Case Reports
and an Experimental Study*

INTERNATIONAL UNIVERSITIES PRESS
New York   New York

First I. U. P. Paperback Printing, 1971
Second I.U.P. Paperback Printing, 1978

CONTENTS

HYPNOTHERAPY: A SURVEY OF THE LITERATURE

FOUR CASE STUDIES

ACKNOWLEDGMENTS

The preparation of this survey of the literature on hypnotherapy was made financially possible by a grant from The Josiah Macy, Jr. Foundation, but to the Director of The Macy Foundation, Dr. Frank Fremont-Smith, we are indebted for far more than financial aid.

The cooperative activity of the group in which we work, The Menninger Foundation staff, was indispensable in this undertaking. Special thanks are due Dr. Karl A. Menninger and Dr. Robert P. Knight, who have consistently encouraged and helped us in all of the research on hynosis in which we are engaged.

We are indebted also to Dr. David Rapaport, Director of Research for The Menninger Foundation, for his many helpful suggestions.

We appreciate the assistance of our former colleague, Dr. Frederick J. Hacker, who contributed to the review of literature included in this survey.

To Miss Clara Louise Meckel, Librarian of The Menninger Foundation, we give thanks for her aid in locating and obtaining all of the references cited.

Other than the authors, the most active participant in the preparation of this manuscript has been Miss Charlotte Ellis, who has devoted great care and energy not only to the secretarial but also to the organizational aspects of preparing the survey. We should like to express our deep gratitude for her part in this work.

THE AUTHORS

PREFACE

This monograph was originally published by the Josiah Macy, Jr. Foundation in 1944 as one volume of its *Review Series* and distributed as part of its wartime service to psychiatrists and psychologists in the armed forces. Since that time, we have continued to receive a steady stream of requests for copies from interested civilians. We have been reluctant to undertake a commercial edition of this survey because we had hoped to delay further publication of our work on hypnosis until such a time as we felt prepared to include the results of our current research. However, we finally decided on this edition, adding two appendices. The first consists of four previously published case studies issuing from the research in hypnotherapy being conducted at the Menninger Foundation under grants from the Macy, New York, and Hofheimer Foundations. The second is a report of an experimental investigation using hypnosis by one of the authors (M.B.). We are indebted to the editors of *The Bulletin of the Menninger Clinic* for permission to reprint the first three of the case studies, and to the editors of *The American Journal of Orthopsychiatry* for permission to reprint the fourth.

INTRODUCTION

It appears from the volume of recent publications in professional journals, and even in popular magazines, that the current attitudes toward hypnosis include a fundamental acceptance of the phenomenon itself as a datum to be investigated by rational scientific methods. However, it has seemed to us that this acceptance is accompanied by a great deal of confusion on every aspect of the problem, and in particular on the role of hypnosis in a rational psychotherapy.

Our discussion will present in the first chapter a brief review of the development of hypnotherapy; in this historical section, we shall attempt to show that the therapeutic applications of hypnosis have usually reflected an implied or a stated psychopathology. In the second chapter we shall summarize the specific methods used to induce hypnosis; this will be a detailed presentation constructed with the aim of providing an outline of procedure for those who might be interested in trying to use some form of hypnotherapy. The third chapter will consist of a short discussion of the factors involved in hypnotic susceptibility, and the techniques which have been used to increase it. In the fourth chapter the most important types of hypnotherapy will be presented and illustrated; this chapter includes the various therapeutic approaches, types of cases treated, indications and contraindications for each, and a discussion of the supposed dangers of hypnotherapy. A fifth chapter on current theories of hypnosis will follow, and we shall conclude with a brief evaluation of the present status of hypnotherapy.

This review will be devoted largely to a discussion of the work done in hypnotherapy during the last fifty years. The investigations before that have been amply summarized by others (3) (28). Although we do not believe that our survey exhausts the recent literature on hypnotherapy, we have tried to select from over twelve-hundred titles those which seemed to contribute most to the problem. The bibliography has been selected with an eye not only to pertinence but also to availability.

HYPNOTHERAPY

A SURVEY OF THE LITERATURE

CHAPTER ONE

THE HISTORICAL DEVELOPMENT
OF HYPNOTHERAPY

It is the purpose of this opening chapter to trace briefly the historic roots of hypnotherapy, in order to show first the persistence of therapeutic applications of hypnosis, and secondly, the manifold attempts to rationalize these applications in some systematic way which would link the therapy with the presumed etiology of the illness. The frames of reference into which the phenomenon of hypnosis has been placed range from the strictly religious systems of the Egyptians, the Persians, and the Hindus, to the most sophisticated theories of present-day psychology.

The theoretical constructs developed to explain the phenomena and to guide the therapeutic applications of hypnosis have evolved along a fairly consistent line; they have moved from a belief in the exclusive importance of physical or physiological processes to a recognition of the significance of psychological factors, and recently include some tentative efforts to achieve, at least in theory, a synthesis of the two. Except for those clinicians who have used hypnosis as a tool without reference to any psychopathology, the specific therapeutic applications have been clear reflections of the theoretical system held to by the therapist.

To date, no satisfactory formulation has been reached. It is our belief that the curious disparity which exists between the rich empirical observations of hypnotherapy, and the primitive state of our understanding of them, is intelligible only as a reflection of the difficulties in the exploration of hypnosis, and of the youthfulness of the science of psychology. We feel, therefore, that the theoretical systematizations that have been attempted thus far are perforce inadequate, but that at present we are in a somewhat better position to evaluate these attempts in the light of the investigations of Freud and his followers.

It is well known that the first effort to bring hypnotherapy within the realm of science was made by Anton Mesmer during the eighteenth century. In line with the dominant scientific interest of his day, he attempted to erect a psychopathology based on disturbances of the "universal fluids" in which man and all the planets are immersed, his cures being mediated through the power of "magnets". Apparently he believed that the iron rods to which his patients held firmly during the seances were the immediate source of the therapeutic power, although he did regard "magnetism" as a human emanation. The next important historical step occurred when the "mesmerists" split among themselves, one group seeking a scientific or rational basis for mesmeric phenomena, the other devoting themselves to developing "mesmerism" as an aspect of clairvoyance. After Mesmer's death, only a few scattered individuals, mainly in Germany and in England, continued these investigations.

The major turning point in the history of hypnotherapy occurred during the fifth decade of the nineteenth century, when James Braid (2), an English doctor and himself at first an arch-skeptic, devoted himself to a re-examination of the so-called "mesmeric phenomena". At first, Braid attempted to consider these as strictly neurophysiological occurrences, and accordingly his therapeutic efforts were regarded by him as attempts to "excite" or "depress" the "nervous energy" of the patient. He believed at first that the secret of "mesmerism" was to be discovered by researches in physiological processes. Later he abandoned this position, and stated that the important point was the subjective or psychological character of these phenomena.[1]

[1] It has frequently been claimed by historians (3) (21) (37) that investigators

In his discussion of the evolution of psychotherapy, Janet (20) points out the efforts of all psychotherapists to integrate their findings within some larger conceptual system. Speaking of the eternal efforts of man to effect intelligible influences on both his inner and outer worlds, he says: "The forces that he summons to help him were first the gods, then by a natural evolution they became natural forces, but very mysterious forces, acting according to unknown laws analogous, in short, to divine caprice." Thus, the importance of Braid's investigations seems to be his effort to bring the phenomena of hypnotherapy within the frame first of neurophysiology and later of an ill-defined psychology, even as Mesmer had leaned on astronomy in his attempt to go beyond the mere observation of phenomena.

It appears, however, that Braid's work was only a first and tentative step in the direction of wresting the facts of hypnosis from both a vague astronomy and a prescientific and speculative neurophysiology. The bitter and extended struggle between the "physicalists" of Paris, led by Charcot (5), and the "suggestionists" of Nancy, under Liebeault (23) and Bernheim (1), had yet to take place before the issue could become clear-cut. Although the work of Charcot was more experimental than therapeutic, and his observations were limited to twelve hysterics at the Salpetriere Clinic (3), his prestige as a neurologist and his emphasis on the tangible made him a formidable opponent to those who championed the elusive "psychological factor" in hypnosis. Bramwell (3) and Janet (20) have shown that the Nancy-Paris controversy was essentially a sophisticated revival of the historic struggle between Braid and the early mesmerists. Logically this period of debate was unnecessary, but historically it was inevitable. Bramwell says:

"All the old errors, the result of ignoring mental influences, are once more revived. Medicines are again

---

like Bertrand, the Abbe Faria, and others had anticipated Braid, but inasmuch as it was Braid who elaborated this psychological view and re-christened the technique "hypnosis", he is usually given the credit.

alleged to exercise an influence from within sealed
tubes. The physical and mental conditions of one
subject are stated to be transferable to another, or
even to an inanimate object. It is useless to enter into
any arguments to refute these statements; for this
would be needlessly repeating the work of Braid.
Indeed, in many instances, their absurdity renders
argument unnecessary: for example when a sealed
tube containing laurel-flower water was brought near
a Jewish prostitute, she adored the Virgin Mary! From
this it might be inferred that different religious beliefs
were represented by different nerve centers, and that
these could be called into action by appropriate physical stimuli."[2]

In the context of this dispute during the classical period of
hypnosis in the '90's, Bernheim's concept of suggestion was a
more meaningful and less pallid notion than its current use
implies. He used the term "suggestion" to stress that the essential mechanisms at work in hypnosis are psychological rather
than physical. This was of crucial importance while the battle
raged; but since the victory of the "suggestionists", the concept of suggestion has lost its impact as a differentiating idea
and has become a shallow cover-all behind which our ignor-
ance of the specific psychological mechanisms hides. Even the
layman no longer supposes that hypnosis is a function of medicines in sealed tubes; he "knows" it is "merely a matter of
suggestion". This was the temporary blind alley into which
the triumph of the psychological approach led. It had been
proved that the stubborn facts of hypnosis could not be fitted
into a physiological frame of reference, but there was as yet
not even a semblance of an organized set of psychological
concepts into which to integrate these facts. Accordingly, the
wild enthusiasm accorded hypnosis during the last two decades
of the nineteenth century waned. Janet (21) says in this connection:

"What was it that the school of Nancy put in place
[2] (3) p. 300.

of this fine dream? A few vague assertions on suggestibility and credulity that could not be discussed or understood without going into the new studies of psychology. But psychology, considered a confused mixture of literature and ethics, had no standing in the school of medicine, and indeed it is a question whether psychology as it was at that period deserved to be more studied by physicians. It may be added that the enthusiastic exaggerations of the hypnotists had brought about the random application of hypnotism in all sorts of disease, without any indication of its fitness, and that the usual results were meaningless or absurd."

The subsequent history of hypnotherapy is largely a record of the attempts of various individuals to use hypnosis in psychotherapy and to formulate a systematic psychopathology within which to operate. Although it might be said that from the beginning the attempt to fit hypnosis into a larger framework inevitably involved some assumptions regarding the etiology of mental illness, the more advanced applications of hypnosis in psychotherapy became much more tightly bound to implicit or stated systems of psychopathology. Most practitioners, however, continued to follow Bernheim in commanding symptom-disappearance "in a clear loud voice" (1). Others drew back in fear from the "irrationalities" of hypnosis, preferring to deal with more readily understandable phenomena and to appeal to the "common sense" of the patient; for the most part, these men rejected hypnosis in their psychotherapeutic practice, and opposed it in their theories. This movement, brought to its most articulate expression by Du Bois (8) and, according to Hart (17), somewhat less puritanically by Dejerine (6), was perhaps the last stand of those psychotherapists who preferred to retain the illusion of "man as a rational animal". Hart has pointed out, however, that even these active opponents of hypnosis and "suggestion" were forced to utilize the patient's emotions as levers in their therapy, whether or not they admitted or even recognized this fact.

Some of the efforts to establish a new rationale for hypnotherapy overlapped in time with the work of Bernheim and Charcot; but inasmuch as the general direction of these attempts was significantly different from the older views, we shall discuss them separately. These were all efforts to meet the gap left by the abdication of the "physicalists", by developing a set of psychological concepts to explain both the origins of mental illnesses and the role of hypnosis in their treatment. We shall reserve extended discussion of current theories for a later chapter, and mention them only briefly here in order to complete the chronological development.

It is of considerable interest that all these transitional psychopathologies took as their point of departure the fact first elaborated in the work on hypnosis, that mental activity may take place in human beings without their being directly aware of it. The development and elucidation of this fundamental discovery leads to the next important series of struggles in the history of psychotherapy in general and hypnotherapy in particular.

Pierre Janet was one of the first who tried to establish links between etiology and therapy (21). Proceeding from his clinical observation and the results of experimental hypnosis, he developed his well-known theory of "dissociation". At first he drew simply on the facts of hypnotic hypermnesia, and on his observations of clinical syndromes in which there appeared to be a "split" or a "disaggregation of consciousness". Later (20) he accounted for hypnotic phenomena and for pathological states (fugues, amnesias, hysterical signs) by ascribing both to a weakening of the "mental synthesis" of the individual. He believed that mental illness was always such a lack of synthesis, and that this represented a more or less reversible state of emotional "bankruptcy". According to him, this weakness made possible the splitting off of certain mental contents from the mainstream of personal consciousness. He tried to give this theory a greater specificity by suggesting that once the weakness existed, those mental contents charged with "strong emotion" would be the more likely to dissociate themselves (20). Janet's complete psychopathology was an elaborate analogy between the human psyche and a great budgetary system. Thus, the aim of all psychotherapy was to restore solvency where bankruptcy had led to dissociation or to excessively costly psychic expenditure. If the difficulty lay in the fact that the patient's "debits" were greater than his "credits", it followed that attempts should be made either to institute economies or to provide new forms of "psychic income". Hypnosis could be applied in either way. The recovery of a dissociated traumatic memory was "an economy through liquidation", whereas direct suggestion was an attempt to strengthen the resources of psychically impoverished patients; they were particularly receptive to such "contributions" while in hypnosis, itself a state of weakened synthesis or "dissociation". Janet was an acute observer and an earnest thinker, but his psychopathology still lacked the nuclear elements of a dynamic psychology; his application of hypnotherapy was accordingly limited. Zilboorg (37) says of him: "Janet actually used the word 'unconscious', seemingly ascribing to it the value of a truly dynamic psychological factor, but he stood before his own excellent description and failed to draw the consequences."

The "consequences" for a dynamic psychopathology were drawn by Sigmund Freud as a direct result of his applications of hypnotherapy in collaboration with Joseph Breuer (4). The latter had discovered the fact that in hypnosis a significant memory might be re-lived, and that this "discharge" of emotion had a therapeutic value. His theoretical systematization of these observations was very close to Janet's, although he used a different vocabulary. Freud had watched Charcot, Liebeault, and Bernheim at work and had been impressed. He tried to interest Charcot in Breuer's method of permitting the patient to talk freely and to express deep feeling, but Charcot was indifferent. Janet, independent of Breuer, had made the same innovation with his hypnotized patients (19) but had stopped short of the final implications of his own work.

The critical last step was taken by Freud alone (15). Unlike Janet, he was not content with the belief that ideas are "split off" sheerly as a result of an inherent weakness of the person, or a quantitative deficit of emotional energy. He felt such a split must take place in a less arbitrary, more lawful way. Such a dissociation was for him not a mere lack of cohesion or a mechanical psychic crumbling, but a systematic necessity for the person: the dissociated set of impulses must be qualitatively different from the mainstream of personal consciousness, and must have been purposively "pushed" from awareness in the patient's effort to protect himself from their onslaught. Freud devoted himself to the elaboration and development of this revolutionary finding, and abandoned the exploration of hypnotherapy within this framework. He gradually built the therapeutic techniques of psychoanalysis and, from his observations, the first dynamic psychopathology.

Now, for the first time, there existed the possibility of viewing hypnosis and hypnotherapy as rational phenomena within the conceptual framework of a scientific psychology; but the accidents of history precluded this. The founder of the new set of concepts had stated that "psychoanalysis . . . only began with my rejection of the hypnotic technique" (11). Thus, for a long time after the publication of *Studies in Hysteria* (4) Freud and his followers avoided the therapeutic application of hypnosis, and only a few isolated attempts were made to suggest a psychoanalytic theory of hypnosis. Freud made one such attempt in his effort to integrate the phenomena of hypnosis with his conception of the role of the group-leader and with the fact of "falling in love" (14). Ferenczi (9), Schilder (32) and others formulated provocative but speculative theories based on the idea that hypnosis is essentially "a resuscitation of infantile erotic masochistic adjustments". Both Ferenczi and Schilder tried to accumulate clinical data to substantiate their theories; although they present some interesting evidence it seems clear that a good deal more will be necessary before a well-founded theory is possible.

Anna Freud (10), following the leads suggested at the outset by her father (4), has tried to show that hypnosis in therapy
seeks to eliminate the ego with all of its defense mechanisms,
thus concealing the resistance of the patient. Although this
view has not been substantiated by clinical observation, it is
at least a hypothesis conceived in the theoretical framework
of a scientific psychology and amenable to empirical check.

It has been unfortunate for the development of hypnotherapy that it was a historical necessity for Freud to reject hypnosis. This left both its practice and theory to those who were
desperately fighting the insights of psychoanalysis. The psychological theories of hypnosis advanced in the first decades of
this century were, with but a few notable exceptions (26),
either variations on Janet's concept of "dissociation" or hybrid
compromises between this view and the Freudian theories.
There were also offered elaborate but highly speculative neurophysiological theories (26) (29) which led to no new advance. The practice of hypnotherapy therefore simply followed one of two old paths: the removal of symptoms by direct
suggestion, or the attempt to remove symptoms by hypnotically
inducing a re-living of one or more specific traumatic episodes.

Typical for this period are the researches of Morton Prince
(29) (30), William McDougall (24) (26), and Boris Sidis
(33) (35) (36). Prince, by far the most conservative of the
three, devoted more of his energy to hypnotic experiment and
exploration than to therapy. He believed like the others in
the existence of mental processes inaccessible to direct awareness, but he insisted on their "logical, orderly" character (31).
He said:

> "Now a word as to my conception of the uncon-
> scious. I conceive the unconscious not as a wild, un-
> bridled, conscienceless subconscious mind, as do some
> Freudians, ready to take advantage of an unguarded
> moment to strike down, to drown, to kill, after the
> manner of an evil genii, but as a great mental mecha-
> nism which takes part in an orderly, logical way in

all the processes of daily life but which under certain
conditions involving particularly the emotion-instincts,
becomes disordered or perverted. We think that in
everyday life we consciously do the whole of our
thinking; but I am inclined to think that our unconscious self does most of our thinking, and that we
simply select from the ideas furnished by the unconscious those which we believe are best adapted to the
situation; that our problems are much more solved
by the unconscious than by the conscious. I regard
the normal unconscious as a logical, orderly mind,
playing an important part in everyday life. Therefore,
as I see it, this conception of unconscious ideas is fundamental, and not the libido, although the instincts
play a tremendous role in carrying, by the force of
their conative impulses, ideas to fruition and setting
up conflicts between opposing ideas with resulting
disharmony."

This notion of a dissociated consciousness, in essence similar to that of consciousness as we ordinarily think of it, actually
goes back to the early discoveries of (so-called) unconscious
processes by workers in hynosis (16) who felt they had proved
their existence by showing that an arithmetical problem could
be solved without the subject having any awareness of this
process. The belief in the essentially rational nature of the
unconscious necessarily leads to an over-rationalistic application of hypnosis in therapy, and completely neglects the role
of instinctual strivings, as well as the nature of symptom-devel-
opment and defense mechanisms. Prince's theoretical position
was very close to that of Janet; McDougall, on the other hand,
while rejecting violently what he termed the "pan-sexuality"
of the Freudians, represented an important advance in that
his concept of the unconscious included a recognition of the
existence of purposive strivings. He developed an independent
psychology, firmly rooted in a belief in the importance of instinctual drives; his therapeutic applications of hypnosis were
thus less academic than those of Prince. Sidis, too, although
holding to a belief in "disaggregations of consciousness", was

closer to a dynamic position. None the less, he launched bitter and scathing denunciations of psychoanalysis, and built his own psychology and psychopathology largely on the "instinct of fear" (36). His most important contribution perhaps lies in his distinction between therapies employing "direct" and "indirect" suggestion (34). He regarded as "indirect suggestion" the use of trickery and deception in therapy (the use of placebos, faradic brushes, and the like). In contrast to this he described the "direct suggestion" of hypnosis, which may be successful in the absence of faith or of credulity. Thus he attacks the nebulous concept of "suggestion", and explores the possibility of giving it some specificity. The implications of this view for the practical applications of hypnotherapy are self-evident.

Since the work of these men during the first decades of this century, little systematic effort has been made to understand hypnosis as a rational phenomenon or to develop it as a tool of psychotherapy within the frame of our modern psychology. Many investigators have tried to do both when dealing with circumscribed experimental or clinical problems; but aside from the work of Schilder and Kauders (32), summarized by them in 1927, there has been no comprehensive statement of the role of hypnosis in modern psychotherapy.

We have seen that hypnotherapy has undergone a historical evolution which has reflected the history of the science of psychology and the development of psychopathology, and that the therapeutic applications have been a direct expression of these. The attempt to understand hypnosis in terms of physical forces or neurophysiological processes failed; this position gave way to an approach which has emphasized psychological factors which we are only now beginning to understand. A synthesis of these positions has seemed impossible. However, the current researches on mechanical adjuvants to hypnotherapy, and on the relationship between drug and hypnotic states, suggests that an integration may finally be achieved.

We have omitted in this chapter many of the great names

in the history of hypnotherapy, because our aim has been not to record the clinical achievements of hypnotherapy, but the significant theoretical developments which altered clinical practice.

CHAPTER TWO

METHODS OF INDUCING AND TERMINATING HYPNOSIS

The induction of the hypnotic state is, in its essence, a simple procedure. Although the literature offers no unequivocal answer to the question, "What factors are the sine qua non of hypnosis?" one can say that most methods of induction include the following elements: a) the limitation of sensory intake and motor output; b) the fixation of attention; c) the repetition of monotonous stimulation; d) the setting up of an emotional relationship between therapist and subject.

It has been argued by Hull (57), Young (84) and others that no one of these factors is prerequisite in order to produce phenomena ordinarily regarded as "hypnotic". Although further research into the nature of hypnosis may show these factors to be unnecessary trappings, it remains a fact that most standard induction procedures involve them. There have been mechanical, chemical, and psychological aids introduced into the process, and these have been minutely catalogued (41) (67). We shall restrict this discussion therefore to a presentation of classic, standard techniques in current use, and shall add a presentation of those adjuvants not previously summarized.

Workers in the field generally agree that a discussion preliminary to the induction is prerequisite. The therapist elicits from the patient his preconceptions and fears regarding hypnosis, and reassures him on one or more of several standard prejudices: that he will not be exposed as a "weakling" should he prove to be a good subject, nor will he be deprived of his "will", or be forced to do anything that will humiliate or frighten him, or lose consciousness at any time, or run the risk of remaining in hypnosis forever. (The completely groundless belief that it is harder to terminate than to induce hypnosis is extremely common.) He is told that, on the contrary, only people of good intelligence and well-developed "will"—in the sense that they can concentrate well—are hypnotizable. If the patient is very anxious for the hypnosis to be successful, he is asked to adopt an attitude of calm detachment insofar as possible, since over-eagerness appears to hinder relaxation. If the patient has undue anxiety regarding the possibility of posthypnotic amnesia, the therapist agrees to let him recall all of his experiences. It is often helpful when using the standard "sleeping method" to discuss hypnosis with the patient as a phenomenon analogous to sleep: he may be told that hypnosis is a kind of sleep in which communication with one person (the hypnotist) remains; this may be compared to the normal phenomenon of a sleeping mother awakened by a faint cry from her infant though louder noises leave her undisturbed, or by a fireman who is awakened only by a particular arrangement of bell signals. When the patient considers hypnosis as a condition allied to sleep, he finds more understandable the hallucinatory experiences, amnesias, and motor helplessness characteristic of deep hypnosis.

The particular variety of doubts raised by the patient is dependent on his intelligence and sophistication; a skillful therapist adapts himself to the needs of the patient in this as in any other psychotherapy, setting up in this initial interview an inter-personal "atmosphere" of sympathy and trust. Often, time can be saved if the therapist assures the patient in advance that no hypnotic phenomena will occur if he decides to try the experiment of pitting his "will" against that of the therapist. When the patient has been given ample opportunity to voice his qualms, he may be told approximately what to expect. It is usually a surprise to the patient to hear that most people are hypnotizable *to some degree,* rather than "either

you are or you aren't". In order to forestall a feeling of inadequacy or failure in the patient, the therapist should describe
in approximate terms the great range of hypnotizability in
people. He may tell the patient that some people feel only a
great lethargy at first, but that some shortly are unable to
open their eyes; and that some very quickly experience a complete immobility, and may develop anesthesias. In general
terms the stages of hypnosis are described[3] as a continuum
extending from a generalized bodily relaxation to somnambulism (the latter usually designating a complete posthypnotic
amnesia and/or the ability to have hallucinatory experiences).

When the therapist is satisfied that he has established a fairly
good pre-hypnotic rapport, and has made the subject comfortable on a couch or in an easy-chair in a semi-darkened room,
he proceeds to attempt to induce hypnosis in one of several
ways: 1. The "sleeping method"; 2. Drug hypnosis; 3. "Hypnoidization"; 4. "Waking hypnosis".

1. The "Sleeping Method"[4]

Before the hypnosis is attempted a number of maneuvers
are often carried out, to serve as an introduction. The Kohnstamm phenomenon is a good beginning (81). The patient is
asked to stand sidewise against a wall and to press the back
of his flexed wrist against it as firmly as possible, while keeping
his eyes closed. This is continued for about one minute, the
therapist exhorting the patient all the while to "press with all
your might, press with your shoulder muscles, your upper arm
muscles, press till you tremble from the strain". When the time
is up the patient is asked to step away from the wall and stand

[3] There is no general agreement, either in the classical or modern literature, on
the precise succession of "stages" of hypnosis. It appears that there exist great
individual differences in this progression, and that no strictly uniform patterns
have been established. Recently Friedlander and Sarbin (51), Davis and Husband (45) and others have attempted to establish quantitative scales of hypnotizability on which subjects may be ranked. However, the fact of individual
differences, as well as the difficulty of establishing a standardized technique of
induction, limits the value of these. A sample scale is shown in Table 1.

[4] This will be a detailed description given with the aim of providing a guide
for those who for the first time attempt to hypnotize patients.

TABLE 1.

THE DAVIS HYPNOTIC SUSCEPTIBILITY TEST (51)

DEPTH	SCORE	OBJECTIVE SYMPTOM
INSUSCEPTIBLE	0	
HYPNOIDAL	1	
	2	Relaxation
	3	Fluttering of lids
	4	Closing of eyes
	5	Complete physical relaxation
LIGHT TRANCE	6	Catalepsy of eyes
	7	Limb catalepsies
	10	Rigid catalepsies
	11	Anesthesia (glove)
MEDIUM TRANCE	13	Partial amnesia
	15	Posthypnotic anesthesia
	17	Personality changes
	18	Simple posthypnotic suggestions
	20	Kinesthetic delusions; complete amnesia
DEEP TRANCE	21	Ability to open eyes without affecting trance
	23	Bizarre posthypnotic suggestions
	25	Complete somnambulism
	26	Positive visual hallucinations, posthypnotic
	27	Positive auditory hallucinations, posthypnotic
	28	Systematized posthypnotic amnesias
	29	Negative auditory hallucinations
	30	Negative visual hallucinations, hyperesthesias

with arms relaxed and hanging at his sides. In the majority of people, the arm in question will rise spontaneously in the air, often even to a 90° angle. The surprised patient is told that this feeling of relaxation and spontaneous movement of a limb is the kind of relaxation and feeling of surrender to external forces that he should attempt to adopt in the hypnotic induction.

Tests of "suggestibility" may then be carried out. Although there is no established relationship between these and hypnotizability, they often serve as good transition. The patient is told to stand with heels and toes together, head forward and eyes closed; to imagine that his body is an upright board hinged to his feet, which he is to imagine as a board at right angles to his body; and that he will feel a force pressing against his forehead and forcing him backward, but that he is not to try to prevent himself from falling since the therapist will stand behind to catch him. The hypnotist then repeats in many variations: "You are falling, you are moving back, you feel as if there were a force pressing again your forehead." If this method is successful, the patient is then asked to try progressively harder to prevent himself from falling, the therapist insisting all the time that he cannot. When it becomes clear that the patient if allowed to exert more effort will be able to prevent himself from falling, the attempt is abandoned. Naturally, one must be practiced and alert to detect this point.

Another introductory procedure is to have the patient sit with arms outstretched before him and fairly close together, with his eyes closed; he is told to picture a toy balloon resting on his hands; the therapist then repeats, with many variations, that as the balloon rises the patient's arms will rise. In most instances, there will be at least a slight elevation. He is now told to picture the balloon descending and that, as he does so, his arms will gradually fall. He is then instructed to picture the balloon motionless, and that his right arm will go up and his left arm down.

These techniques are called tests of "suggestibility", but it is probable that they represent the same phenomena induced by the method of waking hypnosis, described later in this chapter. Any simple motor suggestion can, of course, be substituted for those given here.

The balloon-rising test is carried out with the patient seated in a comfortable chair; and the procedure may continue from here, though some patients relax more easily lying on a couch. An anxious patient is usually more comfortable sitting up. At this point the therapist usually employs some technique of ocular fixation, accompanied in the "sleeping method" by suggestion of drowsiness, relaxation and heaviness.

Bernheim in 1884 (40) described his procedure as follows:

"I say, 'Look at me and think of nothing but sleep. Your eyelids begin to feel heavy, your eyes tired. They begin to wink, they are getting moist, you cannot see distinctly. They are closed.' Some patients close their eyes and are asleep immediately. With others, I have to repeat, lay more stress on what I say, and even make gestures. It makes little difference what sort of gesture is made. I hold two fingers of my right hand before the patient's eyes and ask him to look at them, or pass both hands several times before his eyes, or persuade him to fix his eyes upon mine, endeavoring at the same time to concentrate his attention upon the idea of sleep. I say, 'Your lids are closing, you cannot open them again. Your arms feel heavy, so do your legs. You cannot feel anything. Your hands are motionless. You see nothing, you are going to sleep.' And I add in a commanding tone, 'Sleep'. This word often turns the balance. The eyes close and the patient sleeps or is at least influenced.

"I use the word sleep in order to obtain as far as possible over the patient a suggestive influence which shall bring about sleep or a state closely approaching it; for sleep properly so called does not always occur. If the patients have no inclination to sleep and show no drowsiness, I take care to say that sleep is not essential; that the hypnotic influence, whence comes the benefit, may exist without sleep; that many patients are hypnotized although they do not sleep.

"If the patient does not shut his eyes or keep them shut, I do not require them to be fixed on mine, or on my fingers, for any length of time, for it sometimes happens that they remain wide open indefinitely, and instead of the idea of sleep being conceived, only a rigid fixation of the eyes results. In this case, closure of the eyes by the operator succeeds better. After keeping them fixed one or two minutes, I push the eyelids down, or stretch them slowly over the eyes, gradually closing them more and more and so imitating the process of natural sleep. Finally I keep them closed, repeating the suggestion, 'Your lids are stuck together; you cannot open them. The need of sleep

becomes greater and greater, you can no longer resist.'
I lower my voice gradually, repeating the command,
'Sleep', and it is very seldom that more than three
minutes pass before sleep or some degree of hypnotic
influence is obtained. . . .

" . . . I sometimes succeed by keeping the eyes
closed for some time, commanding silence and quiet,
talking continuously, and repeating the same for-
mulas; 'You feel a sort of drowsiness, a torpor; your
arms and legs are motionless. Your eyelids are warm.
Your nervous system is quiet; you have no will. Your
eyes remain closed. Sleep is coming, etc.' After keeping up this auditory suggestion for several minutes,
I remove my fingers. The eyes remain closed. I raise
the patient's arms; they remain uplifted. We have induced cataleptic sleep."

The importance of keeping a steady, monotonous flow of
"patter" is not clear from this account. It has been our experience, and that of other workers (48), that the average
neurotic who comes for help is not hypnotized to any significant degree within three minutes. Usually, several sessions
of from fifty minutes to an hour-and-a-half are required to induce a deep hypnosis. Erickson (48) has emphasized that, in
many instances, one can expect success only after several hours
of patient, non-routinized effort, with single sessions often
lasting three or four hours.

It is of interest to compare with the original a modern, fairly
standard edition of the "sleeping method", published fifty-
seven years after Bernheim's *Suggestive Therapeutics*. Kraines
(60), whose summary of hypnotherapy is one of the best in
current psychiatric texts, describes the procedure as follows:

"I want you to relax. Relax every part of the body.
Now when I pick up your hand I want it to fall as a
piece of wood without any help from you. (The
examiner then picks up the hand and lets it drop to
the couch.) No, you helped raise the hand that time;
just let it be so relaxed that you have no power over
it. (The test is repeated as often as is necessary for the

patient to learn to let it drop.) That's the way. Now relax your legs the same way; just let them be limp. Now take a deep breath and let it out slowly. Now concentrate on your toes. A warm sensation starts in the toes and sweeps up your legs, abdomen, chest, into your neck. Now relax your jaws. Relax them more, still more. Now your cheeks; now your eyes. Your eyes are getting heavier and heavier. You can hardly keep them open. Soon they will close. Now smooth out the wrinkles in your forehead. Good. Now make your mind a blank. Allow no thoughts to enter. Just blank. You see a blackness spreading before you. Now sleep. Sleep. Sleep. Sleep. Your entire body and mind are re-laxed,—sleep, sleep. (This phrase is repeated several times in a soft and persuasive voice.) Your sleep is becoming deeper, still deeper. You are in a deep, deep, sleep."

There is one striking difference between this description and Bernheim's: here most of the authoritarianism has dropped out. The word "command", extremely common in the older literature (it occurs three times even in the short passage quoted), does not appear even once in the newer version. This is a trend, and not the result of an accidental choice of illustration. In their excellent discussion of the technique of induction, Schilder and Kauders (73) emphasize a strict avoidance of intimidating the subject, and recommend "calm, firm persuasion". Although it could be argued with justice that a deeper hypnosis might be induced in some individuals by the "technique of terror", this gradual change in tactics is consonant with the development of a rational psychotherapy. On the other hand, the therapeutic success of the old "magnetists" who confidently assured their patients that they had been helped by the vital fluid streaming from the therapist's fingertips, and the analogous phenomenon of faith-cures, give pause to the modern psychotherapist, who is usually embarrassed by such irrationalities and is accordingly unable to use any approach which frankly appeals to a primitive layer of the patient's psyche. Some of the modern Germans like Winkel (83) recommend such appeals with unsophisticated patients.

These accounts of Bernheim and Kraines are only the skeleton of the therapist's talk to the patient. These paragraphs can be read in several minutes, but the effort to hypnotize a patient may last an hour or longer. The hypnotist has to repeat his formulae in many ways and many times. But further, he must adapt his remarks to the patient's personality, insofar as he understands it from prehypnotic contacts. He must decide whether to adopt an attitude of unquestionable authority, betraying no hint that he doubts the effectiveness of his suggestions; an intellectual approach in which he explains everything he does; an emotional approach in which he may utilize a patient's particular need for sympathy, comfort, and security; or a passive approach in which he reiterates his ineffectiveness except insofar as he is given authority by the subject, who is led to feel that he is "doing all this" himself. Many other variants in attitude are possible, of course.

In general, in the early phases of attempting induction, the patient should be discouraged from speaking. A patient will often say, "But that's my trouble, I just can't relax" when the hypnotist says, "Now you are relaxing." The reply should be: "Just sit quietly and comfortably and you will find that you will be able to relax more and more," and so forth.

It is difficult to know when one should first challenge the patient, by way of testing his hypnotizability. The general rule is never to challenge unless one is sure that the suggestion will be successful. Naturally, hypnotists vary much in their own temperaments, so that one will challenge early and peremptorily, while another will advance cautiously by small steps.

A first challenge may best be made with regard to the heaviness of an arm. The patient is told that the arm will become progressively heavy. Variations and amplifications of the following formula are used:

> "Your right arm will become very heavy. The heaviness begins in the shoulder, flows down your upper arm to your elbow, then down the forearm to your

> wrist, then into your hand, and then into the fingers, into each individual finger, the thumb, the index finger, the third finger, the fourth finger, and the fifth finger. You will imagine that your arm is turning to lead, beginning at the shoulder, passing down the upper arm to the elbow, and so forth. You feel as if your arm were bound down to the arm of the chair. In your imagination you see steel bands passing over your wrist and your elbow, binding your arm to the chair. You feel that a great suction keeps your arm stuck to the chair, that heavy weights are pressing it down. You will find that it is more and more difficult for you to will to move your arm, and the harder you try the more difficult it will be."

This last phrase, actually a variation of Coué's "law of reverse effort" (44), seems to be peculiarly effective and should be frequently repeated.

If at any time during this attempt the patient shows anxiety, the vigor of the suggestions should be toned down. The patient may also be told that this loss of the ability to move his arm is not a necessary feature of hypnosis, that it might have been suggested that his arm would be unusually light, but that "we are working with the heaviness now".

When the hypnotist feels in a position to challenge the patient, he tells him to try to raise his arm at the count of (say) seven, and that "the harder you try the more difficult it will be". Further suggestions are gauged by the success of this one. It is important to get an admission of at least *some* heaviness, so that the hypnotist has his "foot in the door" and can suggest progressively more. In a completely successful suggestion the patient cannot move his arm at all. Any contraction of the flexors is counteracted by an equally strong or stronger contraction of the extensors. The arm becomes stiff, may tremble with strain, but will not move. The more evidence of strain without success, the more encouraged the hypnotist can be. A cooperative patient anxious to succeed can get lost in the borderland between a feeling of inability despite conscious effort and a lack of trying because of desire to please. Usually the latter will be seen in the absence of strain and stiffening of the arm, but this is not always the case. Again the hypnotist must know just when to challenge a patient who is not trying to exert greater and greater effort; but this can be learned only through practice.

It is sometimes wise, before the challenge to raise the arm, to have the patient press down against the arm of the chair very firmly for a few seconds, as though to give him the cue for what should happen; he is of course not told what this is for.

From here on the progress of the induction is an attempt to produce deeper and deeper hypnotic phenomena, utilizing the same general principles described in producing inability to raise the arm, and progressing by the smallest steps necessary in the hypnotist's opinion to permit him to challenge with fair certainty of success. In most subjects, of course, the time soon comes when one can go no deeper. When suggested inability to move the arm is almost or entirely successful, inability to open the eyes is next suggested. The arm is chosen before the eyes because it is much easier to work with degrees of lifting the arms than with degrees of opening the eyes; and opening them in the face of the suggestion to be unable to do so, is often seriously disruptive to the whole procedure and shakes the patient's confidence. It is often wise to have the patient first squeeze his eyes shut as tightly as possible, and to use the phrase "tight until they tremble". Once the hypnotist has challenged the subject, he should not merely sit quietly but leap in with his counter-suggestions at once, saying, "You see that you are unable to do so, your best efforts only make it more difficult," and so on.

After these muscular phenomena are successful, one can turn to suggesting anesthesia. It is considerably easier to produce a hypesthesia than an anesthesia, so that at first one should only suggest a dulling of sensation and not attempt to go beyond this unless successful. The back of the hand is a convenient place to use, and the testing may be carried out with the sharp and dull ends of a pin.

The hypnotic phenomenon usually considered next in degree of depth is amnesia. The immediate amnesia is that produced within the hypnotic session. The patient is first told that alterations in memory are possible in the hypnotic state, that they are important in therapy particularly because they allow the recovery of buried material, and that, in working with the problem now, the hypnotist will show the subject how material present in the mind may be first accessible to consciousness and then not. This is compared to the everyday experience of knowing something but being unable to say it, having it "on the tip of the tongue". In attemping to produce this immediate amnesia, visual aids are often valuable. In fact, throughout the induction of hypnosis, one should attempt to use colorful, sense-laden figures of speech, because they make the suggestions more vivid and compelling. The subject may be told to imagine a blackboard on which he writes three different words suggested by the hypnotist. He is then told to erase these in his imagination; the words will drop out of his memory so that later, when asked to reproduce them, he will find that he has to grope for them and may indeed be unable to recall them. The hypnotist proceeds for a time with suggestions of relaxation and drowsiness as before, and then returns to the words. As with heaviness of the arm, it is important to get an admission of at least some difficulty with the words, so that one can then build up and insist that this difficulty will grow greater and greater until the words cannot be recalled. When this is successfully achieved, the patient is told that, at the count of a given number, the words will return; and they then do. It is understood of course that when the therapist fails with one of the steps here outlined, it is unlikely that the patient will be susceptible to the next one. This is by no means invariably true, and cases have frequently been reported in which amnesia is obtainable when muscular phenomena are not, and vice versa; but these are not the common results.

If immediate amnesia is successful or approximately so, one may suggest a corresponding degree of posthypnotic amnesia, which is sometimes more easily obtainable. The patient is told that, after awakening, it will seem to him he has been asleep or dreaming and his memory for what has happened will be hazy, or (if, in the hypnotist's opinion, the suggestion appears warranted) that there will be no memory at all of the hypnosis.

As already emphasized, the phenomena described are progressively deeper only in a relative sense, as many variations occur. The one usually obtainable next is the carrying out of a posthypnotic suggestion. This concept is well known, and need not be further defined here. The carrying out of the command is more likely if amnesia for it is suggested, and if the command is "reasonable"—that is, not a bizarre act which would excite unusual attention and be unlike the behavior one might expect from the subject.

Next comes the positive sensory hallucinations; and here, as before, the more patiently, vividly and "reasonably" the suggestions are given, the more likely will they be to succeed.

"Negative hallucinations" are the loss by hypnotic suggestion of the reality of some sensory impression, such as the ability to recognize the presence of a particular person in the room. Such phenomena represent of course a deep stage of hypnosis, and can be carried out with the eyes open and the subject in a "trance state" which to the casual observer may appear to be the behavior of a normal, wide-awake person. It is questionable whether one should make these latter tests of hypnosis in subjects to be treated later by hypnotherapy. Probably one should confine tests to the production of inability to lift the arm and open the eyes; if this is successful, one might see what degree of amnesia could be produced, and there let the matter drop. In the therapeutic situation it is of course always necessary to make it perfectly clear to the patient that a deep hypnosis is not required for therapeutic results. This in fact, as will be seen in subsequent chapters, is consistent with our knowledge of hypnotherapy.

As a technical aid both in inducing hypnosis and in judging its depth, Sargent and Fraser (72) have recommended hyperventilation; they suggest that the increased willingness of the patient to breathe deeply is a sign of his responsiveness. Another good means of deepening the hypnosis is Vogt's "method of fractionation" (78). The patient is hypnotized, "awakened", and then immediately hypnotized again. This may be repeated several times within the same session. The termination of each hypnotic session is brought about in the "sleeping method" by simply telling the patient that at a given signal (e.g., "when I count to five") he will "wake up". It is wise to assure the patient, while he is still in hypnosis, especially during the first few sessions, that he will feel "well and rested, as if he had taken a nap".

All of the progression described may be accomplished in one hour, if the patient is an excellent subject; or it may take much longer. Our own procedure is to work for one hour, and at the end of that time to wake the patient, after telling him that in the next session at the count of ten he will reach the depth reached in the first session and that then the hypnosis can be still further deepened. This is repeated at the end of each session. If the patient has reached the stage of eye-closure, one can say that "by the time I have reached ten, your eyes will have closed". Usually the patient does not return at once to the stage reached in the first session, and some work is necessary to bring him to that stage before one can continue. The time taken to wake a patient without any "after-effects" varies with different subjects and with the degree of practice. If a particular session is followed by a little dizziness, it is wise to take a little longer the next time. Some hypnotists feel that it is necessary to remove every suggestion by careful and detailed counter-suggestion, but it is our experience that general blanket suggestions of well-being and disappearance of the phenomena of the hypnosis are enough.

The "sleeping method" has sometimes been used to induce hypnosis in a group of patients. Wetterstrand (80) used the group technique extensively. Hadfield (54) reports its use with war neuroses. The procedure is essentially the same as in working with the individual patient. In group work, the therapist must rely far more on his authority and on the contagion of emotions than in individual hypnosis, because he cannot adapt himself to individual needs.

2. *Drug Hypnosis*

This is usually a variety of the "sleeping method", the only difference being that chemical means are employed to induce hypnosis when verbal methods have failed, or simply to accelerate it. Bechterew (39) has suggested, in fact, that not only is there a physiological relation between hypnosis and sleep, but that hypnosis, narcosis, and normal sleep comprise a continuum.

If one compares the summaries of drugs used during the nineties—mainly chloroform and Cannabis indica (41)—with the more recent reports, it appears that the only significant change has been in the direction of employing drugs with a more rapid action, the effects of which wear off more quickly and which, on the whole, have less the character of "knock-out drops". This trend has not been clear-cut or consistent, however. Kubie (61) has summarized most of the drugs recently employed in this field; in most instances, he gives specific dosages recommended.

Schilder and Kauders (73) reject the use of chloroform, employed with good success by earlier investigators, and recommend medinal (usual dosage 0.5 to 1 gram with the maximum of 1.5 grams). For a more prompt effect, they suggest between 4 and 12 grams of paraldehyde, doses of over 8 grams being exceptional. With this drug, one must take care to produce the hypnosis quickly, lest the patient attain a depth of slumber which makes him inaccessible.

The best recent discussion of the use of drugs in hypnotherapy is Horsley's (56). He believes with Grinker and
Spiegel (53) that the barbiturates act specifically on the hypothalamic region.[5] Horsley (56) reports his investigations of
nembutal, sodium amytal and particularly sodium pentothal.
Using the last he was able to establish good hypnotic rapport
with eighteen of twenty nurses, and produce hypnotic phenomena (catalepsy, hallucinations, hypermnesia, and so forth)
in many. The production of hypermnesia in narcotic hypnosis
differentiates it from simple narcosis, in which there are varying degrees of drowsiness with confusion, disorientation, and
incoherence. Also in narcotic hypnosis, he was successful in
restoring memories of previous states of narcosis for which the
patient had become amnesic. Horsley recommends the use of
drug adjuvants for patients who have resisted other methods
of induction, for those who are inaccessible (e.g., sodium amytal in catatonic schizophrenics), for mute, agitated or depressed
patients, and for acute war neuroses in the field. It is not
always easy to distinguish between simple narcosis and narcotic hypnosis, if no tests are made beyond that of eliciting
material from the patient. There does not exist in the literature
as yet any crystallization of the significant differentials.

One of the most enthusiastic recent investigations of drug
hypnosis is Brotteaux's work on the use of a compound of
scopolamine and chloralose (or chloral), which he has chris-
tened "scopochloralose" (42). As a result of more than a decade
of work, he maintains that his "scopochloralose" has been successful in inducing a reliable hypnosis where not only verbal
but other drug methods have failed. He has conducted systematic experimentation with normal people in order to estab-

---

[5] Although Grinker and Spiegel tend to the view that the effects of sodium
pentothal are distinct from the phenoma of hypnosis, we mention their recent
monograph in connection with "drug hypnosis" because our own experience
indicates sufficient phenomenal overlapping between the two to make their
monograph a valuable reference for those working with drug hypnosis. Grinker
(52) has recently stated the view that the relationship between states of
narcosis and hypnosis has not yet been clearly defined, and bears further investigation.

lish the relation of the effects of "scopochloralose" to ordinary hypnosis; and he found that in most instances he was able to produce posthypnotic suggestions, amnesias, and hallucinations even where many other induction techniques had been tried without success. He speaks of bringing about a state in which it is possible to "give suggestions to the unconscious" and feels that this accessibility is greatest at the beginning of drug-induced anesthesia. The narcotic hypnosis follows within two to four hours after taking the drug, and verbal hypnotic methods are introduced only after the subject has begun to be drowsy. With patients, therapeutic suggestions or explorations are now begun. The patient is then permitted to sleep for four or five hours, providing—according to Brotteaux—an opportunity for "unconscious rumination". Schilder and Kauders (73) have mentioned this also. He emphasizes that he regards not the drug, but the specific hypnotic investigations and suggestions, as the critical therapeutic agent; and reports many startlingly rapid, permanent cures. It is of interest that, although it was found possible to produce a profound hypnosis in psychotics by using "scopochloralose", they remained completely unresponsive to therapeutic suggestions.

Another recent attempt to establish links between the phenomena of hypnosis and those of narcosis has been made by Stungo (77), working with evipan sodium. He says: "There is no practical distinction between the hypnotized and the narcotized patient." He uses a 10 per cent solution, injected intravenously at the rate of 1 cc. per minute. The patient counts backwards, and usually reaches the proper stage after 1 to 3 cc. Stungo attempts to maintain this level by continuous injection. Horsley (56) has justly criticized the technique of having the patient count backwards as too stereotyped and mechanical. He prefers to carry on a continuous conversation with the patient, and to note the point at which he becomes confused, as well as the nature of this confusion.

Most workers who have employed the methods of "drug hypnosis" agree on certain points of general procedure. For instance, it has been found that, once a deep soporific hypnosis has been attained with the aid of a drug, subsequent hypnoses may be readily induced by verbal methods alone (73) (61). The drug should be dispensed with, whenever possible, to avoid a possible addiction. It has been recommended also that the patient be permitted to "sleep off" the effects of the drug before he returns home, both for his protection and for observation of his reaction by the therapist. This has been found unnecessary, however, with rapidly-acting drugs like paraldehyde or sodium pentothal.

We come now to a consideration of the advantages and disadvantages of the use of drug adjuvants. The advantages lie first in the fact that the response to chemical means of altering states of consciousness is more general than to verbal methods;[6] secondly, any physician may give an intravenous injection and expect some results, without having been trained in the specific techniques of hypnosis. In addition, there are no longer social taboos on the use of "medicine" in treatment, whereas some fear and suspicion of the strictly verbal methods of unvarnished hypnosis still exist. Maclay (65), who has described the use of sodium amytal in "narcoanalysis", feels that this is a point of central importance, and makes it clear that in the administration of this therapy at the Mill Hill Sanitarium no links with hypnotherapy are made. When the practical situation dictates such a severance of the allied methods of hypnosis and narcosis, it seems unnecessary that the therapist sacrifice the accumulated data on hypnotherapy even in his techniques and in his therapeutic approach. Perhaps it is possible to retain the advantage of a greater social acceptance of the use of drugs, without foregoing the orientation provided by the historical development of hypnosis.

One of the primary disadvantages of the use of drugs lies in the danger that the therapy, whether of the suppressive or "uncovering" type, may take on the character of a compart-

---

[6] Hadfield (54) has recently pointed out that this is not always the case; that in some instances verbal methods succeed where drugs have failed.

mentalized or "split-off" experience. Maclay (65) and Grinker (53) have both mentioned the fact that the patient often has amnesia for the period of narcosis. (This difficulty is clearly recognized by Grinker, who attempts to counter with a follow-up of integrative, synthesizing psychotherapy; to a lesser extent, this is done by Maclay also.) The radical physiological alterations in the patient during narcosis make difficult the bridging of this gap, as the patient must often be given benzedrine or some other stimulant in order to keep him awake. Sometimes the patient is accessible only for a short period as he enters the state of narcosis and as he emerges from it, and often he becomes drowsy too soon to make any real contact possible. Another disadvantage of the drug method is the fact that it cannot be repeated—without unfavorable side reactions—as often and at as close intervals as may be indicated.[7] Kubie (61) points out that it is definitely contraindicated "for any debilitated patient and for any patient suffering from severe cardiorespiratory involvement or hepatic disease". As an antidote, 1.5 to 3.0 cc. of a 25 per cent solution of diethyl-nicotinamide intravenously is recommended.

The drug methods have been used more frequently than the verbal in the treatment of the psychiatric casualties of World War II. The reason for this is not entirely clear, although it may be that here again historical accident plays a role, in that most physicians in the neuropsychiatric units have been trained in the administration and use of drugs, and feel more at home with them than with the verbal methods of hypnosis. It is part of the routine medical training of the psychiatrist to give intravenous injections, but it is only by accident or by dint of a special interest that he acquires any knowledge of the techniques of hypnosis. Fisher (49) has pointed out, in addition, some of the emotional "blocks" which may operate; it is his opinion that many inexperienced therapists hesitate to enter into an intense relationship with the patient, and to be con-

[7] Rogerson (69) has attempted to meet this difficulty by using nitrous oxide, which does not carry the hazards of the barbiturates.

fronted by explosive unconscious material. Actually, in some of the therapeutic applications of hypnosis, no such necessity is met; a drug-induced state of hypnosis may be utilized for many different kinds of psychotherapy. Just as with the verbal methods of hypnosis, the end-state may be used to facilitate the suppression of symptoms by direct suggestion; it may be a means of maintaining a calm and prolonged sleep; or it may be used to aid an "uncovering" type of psychotherapy.[8]

3. "Hypnoidization"

Despite the fact that Sidis (74) (75) (76) took great pains to argue that the hypnoidal state is not a variant of hypnosis, the procedure and phenomena are so close to those we call "hypnotic" that we feel justified in including a description of them here. Sidis believed that the hypnoidal state is the most primitive kind of rest-state out of which conditions of waking, normal sleep, and hypnosis have become differentiated. He characterized it as a highly fluid and volatile transitional state, which fluctuates between waking on the one hand and sleep or hypnosis on the other. There are thus "varying degrees of access to the subconscious" (47), and attitudes of "criticism and resistance" are suspended. As with any other induction method, the therapeutic applications have consisted of a variety of methods, including direct suggestion and protracted and intensive investigations of the etiology of the disturbance.

Donley (47), a disciple of Sidis, describes the technique as follows:

> "The patient is asked to close his eyes and keep as quiet as possible, without, however, making any special effort to put himself in such a state. He is then asked to attend to some stimulus such as reading or singing. When the reading is over, the patient with his eyes still shut, is asked to repeat it and tell what came into his mind during the reading, during the repetition, or after it. Sometimes, as when the song

[8] See Chapter Four, on "Therapeutic Applications".

stimulus is used, the patient is simply asked to tell the nature of ideas and images that entered into his mind at this time or soon after."

During this time the patient reclines on a couch in a half-darkened room, very much as in the "sleeping method". There were many variations of this technique. Coriat (46) would read newspaper clippings of indifferent content to his patients, or ask them to attend closely to the ticking of a watch or the beat of a metronome. Sidis (75) regards these hypnoidal states as closer to waking and therefore more "normal" than hypnosis.

Sidis further discusses, as an aspect of the transition between sleep and waking, the "hypnagogic state" in which "dream-hallucinations hold sway". Kubie and Margolin (63) have recently conducted systematic investigations of the production of such "hypnagogic reveries" by use of a physiological method with the aim of securing free associations and early memories. The patient's own breath sounds are picked up by a contact microphone placed against the neck, amplified, and brought back to the patient through earphones. After a short time, the patient gradually falls into a "hypnagogic state". The authors report that this method of induction results in a free and vivid flow of free associations, which gravitates to early experiences of an intensely emotional variety. In a recent article (62) Kubie says:

"The hypnagogic reverie might be called a dream without distortion. Its immediate instigator is the day's 'unfinished business', but like the dream it derives from more remote 'unfinished business' of an entire lifetime as well. The hypnagogic reverie differs from a dream in the fact that there is less elision of the remote and recent past, and far less use of symbolic representation. This would seem to be due to two facts: in the first place, since the reverie does not attempt to say as much as a dream, it does not need to depend upon condensed hieroglyphics to express multiple meanings. In the second place, when the hypnagogic reverie is artificially induced for therapeutic purposes, guilt and anxiety seem to play a less active role than in a dream, with the result that the content of the reverie can come through with less disguise. Whatever the explanation, the consequence is that through the induction of states of hypnagogic reverie, significant information about the past can be made readily and directly accessible, without depending upon the interpretations which are requisite in the translation of dreams."

He points out that "in a number of patients, in whom prolonged analysis had not succeeded in penetrating to the roots of a neurosis, the addition of this technique has proven invaluable", but he feels that further investigation will be necessary before the specific applicability of this method will be known. It is of particular interest that the theoretical frame of reference of these recent studies leans to the physiological aspects of hypnoidal and hypnotic states, with a conscious attempt to minimize personal contact. This revival of interest in the physiological aspects may well serve as a starting point for a genuine synthesis of the historically warring camps, inasmuch as this interest is not considered as independent of, or in contradiction to, the psychological emphasis.

Sidis (76) and Donley (47) have pointed out the advantages of "hypnoidization": it may be used with success with greater numbers of people than classic hypnosis; it is a simpler process; and the word "hypnosis" need not be mentioned to the patient. Sidis reported, moreover, unusual therapeutic success, presumably as a result of the use of this method.

4. "Waking Hypnosis"

The "waking" method of induction developed from the view that sleep and hypnosis are distinct phenomena. From this assumption, it follows that all the standard hypnotic responses may be induced in a patient without any reference to sleep. Although this method is less commonly used than the "sleeping method", we include a discussion of it because it has several distinct advantages. Wells (79) has pointed out that Braid attempted to suppress the word "hypnotism" over a hundred years ago, when he concluded that sleep is not essential to all the phenomena he had previously called "hypnotic"; he tried to substitute the word *monoideism*, but this was never accepted by workers in the field. Wells has reported the development of "waking hypnosis" in great detail, and points out that Bernheim, Lloyd Tuckey, Moll, Forel and others had independently observed and reported the production of hypnotic phenomena in the waking state.

Wells describes his technique of "waking hypnosis" by contrasting it with the usual "sleeping methods". He says that whereas the usual technique includes an explanation in terms of sleep, direct and indirect suggestions of sleep, and an experiencing of drowsiness by the patient, the "waking method" excludes all of these. He suggests that:

> "Examples of involuntary ideo-motor action may be given, such as the tendency of the hand to illustrate a spiral if one is attempting verbal definition of it. Examples of absent-minded actions and of lapses of memory may be given, as illustrations of dissociation in the waking state. Then, without any reference whatever to sleep or to drowsiness one may proceed to an artificial manipulation of the subject's attention so as to produce by direct suggestion the various dissociative effects that one may desire."

After a few preliminary experiments, he usually asks the patient to fix his attention on a simple object—a ring, a fountain pen, a point of light—and repeats to the patient some variation of the following:

> "You must exclude all other thoughts and keep your gaze riveted on this point, eyeballs turned up as though you were looking at the middle of your forehead. Watch it steadily, fixedly, thinking of nothing else. Note every detail so that if I ask you to close your eyes you will be able to picture it as though you were

still looking at it. You will be able to do this only if
you give it your complete attention and literally feel
that you are memorizing it. Watch it closely, try not
to blink. Don't let your gaze shift to right or left . . . "

When the patient seems to have succeeded in fixing his
attention completely on the stimulus and has watched it
steadily for several minutes, he is told:

"Now close your eyes voluntarily as tight as you
possibly can. Tight until they tremble. Tight until
they tremble. It's all right if you have to make a face
in order to do so. Just as tight as you can, eyeballs
turned up, remember, just as if you were still look-
at my fountain pen. Now I'm going to count to seven
and when I reach seven you will find that your eyes
are stuck tight and that the harder you try to open
them, the tighter they stick. Your very effort to open
them will have just the opposite effect. They will be
stuck tight, just as if they were glued. One . . .
two . . . tighter . . . three . . . four . . . five . . .
tighter . . . six . . seven. Now try to open them and
you will find that the harder you try, the tighter they
stick."

If this direct suggestion is successful, and the patient is
convinced that despite his voluntary effort he is unable to
open his eyes, the therapist may proceed to induce the other
muscular contractures in much the same way—e.g., to give the
direct suggestion that if the hands are clasped tightly together they cannot be unclasped, and so on—and then advance
to the other hypnotic phenomena listed in Table 1. If this
first direct suggestion is not immediately successful, the therapist should assure the patient that sometimes it takes a little
longer for these phenomena to appear. Then he should work
with other muscular contractures, and return to eye-closure
later. At the close of the session, as in "sleeping hypnosis",
the patient will come out of the trance at an arbitrarily established signal—such as, "when I say the letters from 'A' to

'G' you will gradually come back to your normal self: at 'A', you will move your feet; at 'B', your arms (and so on); and at 'G', you will open your eyes and feel perfectly normal once again." If therapeutic suggestions have been given, care should be taken to avoid such expressions as, "you will be just the same as when you came in". Although the caution may seem superfluous, this is a frequent technical error.

There exists a close kinship between "waking hypnosis" and the specific techniques of Coué and the "New Nancy School" (44). *We refer here only to the method of induction and not to the therapeutic approach.* Although in his later writings Coué did not use the word "hypnosis" at all, it is clear from the statements of Baudouin (38), his theoretician, that Coué's techniques were historically rooted in hypnosis and that in fact Coué began by "putting his patients to sleep" (44). Direct suggestion in the normal state was characteristic of Coué's later method.

Although it would take us into too great a digression to discuss in detail the historical significance of Coué's "auto-suggestionist" movement, we should like to point out in passing that, like the system of Mary Baker Eddy, it was actually a crude attempt to deal with the dawning recognition that the forces both of illness and recovery lie essentially within the person and not in an external agent.[9] It is a recognition of the power of the unconscious. Thus, Coué's famous little pamphlet, *Self-Mastery Through Conscious Auto-Suggestion,* is sub-titled, "The Conscious Self and the Unconscious Self". On a far more urbane level, Baudouin has explicitly expressed the sympathies of the "New Nancy School" for the work of the psychoanalysts: "Contemporaneously with, but independently of, the idea of psychoanalysis (developed along divergent lines by Breuer and Freud, on the one hand, and by the Zurich school, on the other), the idea of the 'New Nancy School',

---

[9] A more recent investigation along the same line is Salter's work on auto-hypnosis (70) (71). This work differs from the "auto-suggestionist" inquiries in the fact that Salter begins by using a standard "sleeping method".

clearer than the former and more akin to the French spirit, leads us by a path parallel with that opened by psychoanalysis, into the little-known domain of the subconscious, and contributed likewise to the renovation of psychology, medicine, and pedagogy. The two outlooks are complementary."

The essential difference between Coué's method and "waking hypnosis" lies in the fact that whereas Coué restricted his "waking suggestions" to early stages of light hypnosis (mainly contractures), Wells has shown that one may produce by direct suggestion the "characteristic phenomena usually associated with deep sleeping hypnosis". He summarizes its advantages on the basis of his experiments with several hundred subjects. The "waking method" is, according to him, easier to learn and gives less the impression of an occult procedure; it usually takes a significantly shorter time and requires far less effort on the part of the therapist. He has found it to be successful with a larger percentage of subjects than the "sleeping methods".

"Waking hypnosis" may be used either in groups or with individuals. The practical importance of trying to hypnotize twenty people at once, in an effort to pick out the best subjects, will be at once obvious to anyone who has attempted to hypnotize twenty individuals consecutively. In situations where such time and labor-saving techniques are prerequisite (as in the armed forces), group hypnosis seems preferable. Once the best candidates have been chosen, individualized hypnotherapy may be instituted.

We have described the most important variations in techniques of inducing hypnosis. The individual therapist usually develops his own from one or more of these, adapting himself to the needs of each patient, combining techniques where it seems necessary, and varying his approaches even with the same patient. At present we have so little genuine understanding of the specific psychological processes which constitute these various methods that it is as yet difficult to evaluate them. The advocates of each approach offer clinical evidence for the special effectiveness of each technique. It would be important to delineate the ways in which the underlying attitudes of the patient in "sleeping" and "waking" hypnosis differ from each other, and from those in the "hypnoidal state"; and the essential differences between all of these and the attitudes of patients given psychotherapy in the normal state, whether it be the relaxed, uncritical attitude of the analysand or the "conversation" of a patient in standard psychotherapy. Only by a systematic comparison of these states, and of their effect on the course of psychotherapy, will there emerge conclusions regarding the comparative value of these methods.

CHAPTER THREE

SUSCEPTIBILITY TO HYPNOSIS

Before turning to a discussion of the various methods of hypnotherapy we shall deal briefly with the questions that logically precede such a discussion: "Which persons are most susceptible to hypnosis?" and "What are the crucial factors in determining hypnotizability?" The therapist would like to be spared fruitless effort with patients who will probably be refractory and to choose only those known to be responsive to this form of treatment. Unfortunately, no definite answer has been given by the literature, and the average hypnotherapist has his unverbalized "hunches" which he then tests on a more or less trial-and-error basis.

The most complete summary of susceptibility to hypnosis has been made by Bramwell (89) who draws the following conclusions on the basis of reports by many independent investigators: a) From 78 to 97 per cent of the total population are hypnotizable *to some degree.* b) Only 10 to 20 per cent of young adults can achieve the deepest state of hypnosis. c) There is apparently an age factor in hypnotizability—55 per cent of children from seven to fourteen years of age could be hypnotized to the deepest level whereas this was true of only 7 per cent of persons ranging in age from fifty-six to sixty-three. It is extremely difficult, however, to evaluate these figures inasmuch as no standard criteria of hypnosis have been yet devised.

Only a few general characteristics have been agreed upon by most investigators as favorable for the induction of hypnosis. Bramwell has summarized these: a good hypnotic subject has at least "a fair intelligence"; he is usually under fifty years of age; he does not have a severe attention disturbance; and he is, above all, willing to cooperate in the experiment. Erickson (93) believes that cooperativeness is an important characteristic. He says: " . . . any really *cooperative* subject may be . . . (hypnotized) . . . regardless of whether he is a normal person, a hysterical neurotic, or a psychotic schizophrenic patient." Most workers in the field are somewhat less optimistic; they agree, for the most part, that mentally ill persons are significantly more difficult to hypnotize than normals[10] (100) (101) (96) (88), and that it is almost impossible to hypnotize psychotics (91). Voisin (110), Schilder (107), Jenness (98), Flatau (95), and Winkel (115) have, however, reported some success in hypnotizing psychotics. Race, sex, nationality and social class seem to have little or no influence on susceptibility (89).

The attempt to discover what it is that "makes a person go into hypnosis" has thus far been largely restricted to studies of the personality characteristics of the subjects. If "hypnosis" is in part a unique interpersonal *relationship*, it may be that the approach which studies only one aspect of this relationship (namely, the subject himself) is foredoomed to failure. At any rate, the results of studies of good and poor subjects have not yielded any consistent results. We present them only to provide a summary of current hypotheses.

Hull (97) has reported studies that tried without success to establish significant correlations between personality "traits" and hypnotizability. One study by M. M. White (111) reported a positive correlation between "extroversion" and hypnotizability as measured by a "paper-and-pencil" personality inventory but a subsequent investigation by Barry, MacKinnon

---

[10] William Brown is the only consistent opponent of this view. Holding to Charcot's belief in the close similarity between hypnosis and hysteria, he believes that hysterics are especially easy to hypnotize but that they become less hypnotizable as they become cured. .

and Murray (85) who employed the same test did not confirm White's findings. Davis and Husband (92) even found slight though unreliable evidence for a correlation between "introversion" and hypnotic susceptibility. In this same study, they attempted to investigate several other factors in relation to hypnotizability (intelligence, maladjustment, prejudice, and affectivity). They conclude that there is no evidence for Janet's belief that susceptibility is linked with neurotic tendencies and that the only factor that does seem to be related to hypnotizability is that of general intelligence. (They obtained a low positive correlation of .34 between these two variables.)

Another line of approach has been the attempt to correlate the rise and fall of auditory threshold in reverie with hypnotizability. In Morgan's investigation (102) the auditory threshold was obtained and then the patient was told to abandon himself to reverie and day-dreaming. Morgan reports that in schizophrenics the threshold goes up and that in psychoneurotics it goes down during reverie. Every person whose threshold was lowered during reverie and who was tested for hypnotizability could be hypnotized; and not a single one whose threshold was raised could be.

This work issued in an effort to set up constellations in which hypnotizability does or does not appear. In one group, were placed those individuals who can readily lose themselves in day-dreaming and who respond during such a period of reverie to a weaker sensory stimulus than when paying strict attention to the stimulus (lowering of the threshold). Such persons were characterized as having a "dissociative" type of personality and could readily be hypnotized. The other group, who could not be hypnotized, was comprised of persons who cannot abandon themselves to reverie and who respond during such an attempt at day-dreaming only to a more intense stimulus than when paying strict attention to the stimulus (raising of the threshold). They showed a "shattering" of personality rather than a "dissociation".

Jenness and Dahms (98) have since reported, however, that of eight good hypnotic subjects, the auditory thresholds of six rose during reverie. This directly opposed finding causes considerable doubt concerning the utility of this test as an index of hypnotizability. Bartlett's findings (86) also suggest that these liminal changes are not related to clinical types but to fluctuations in certain immediate physiological factors.

Bartlett in another investigation (87) compared the responses to direct suggestion of a group of normals with two patient groups: one, psychoneurotic and the other schizophrenic. There was little difference in the response between the normal and neurotic groups, although the normal subjects tended to respond more positively to the suggestions. It is curious that within the neurotic group the best response came from the "psychasthenics", with the "hysterics" running a poor second. Whereas over 30 per cent of both normal and neurotics reacted positively, this was true only for 16 per cent of the schizophrenics, all of the paranoid group. In the simple hebephrenic and catatonic types, there were no positive responses whatever. Here again, these are only tentative conclusions based on small samples. Similar results, however, were obtained by Williams (114). There is also some clinical evidence for questioning the belief that hysterics are necessarily good hypnotic subjects. H. C. Miller (100) agrees with Moll (101) and Forel (96) that the hysteric is the "most difficult to influence".

The most frequent criticism of all of the above mentioned studies has been that the instrument employed to arrive at "personality characteristics" has never been sufficiently sensitive to tap any significant aspects of the subject's personality. Recently, there have been several investigations conducted which have utilized the "projective test" methods on good and poor hypnotic subjects. Responses on the Rorschach Inkblot test[11] were analyzed in relation to hypnotizability by Sarbin

[11] In this test the subject is asked to look at an inkblot and to tell what "it might

and Madow (106) and by Brenman and Reichard (90). The former found a positive correlation between the "whole-detail ratio" and hypnotizability. This was not confirmed by the latter who conclude: "Although our results suggest that 'ego-centric affective responsiveness' may be involved, it would seem that the factor of 'free-floating anxiety' is of even greater importance in hypnotizability. Thus, if one assumes with Rorschach that responses purely to color or even to a combination of color and form are characteristic of ordinarily 'suggestible' persons, it would appear that there does not necessarily exist a one-to-one relationship between hypnotizability and every-day suggestibility. That is to say, "suggestibility alone, as Rorschach understood it, appears insufficient to make the individual a good hypnotic subject."

Yet another (and, in the opinion of the present reviewers, more promising) application of projective techniques has been the use of the Thematic Apperception test.[12] R. W. White (112) found that the average correlation between the actual rank order of hypnotizability and the guessed rank order of several judges, who estimated the probable hypnotizability of each subject on the basis of his "hypnosis story" was .34. The correlation was higher (.50) where the judges were better acquainted with the problems of hypnosis. White concludes:

> "Though the procedure was too crude, and the subjects too few, to warrant more than a tentative generalization, it seems indicated that stories which subjects make up on the theme of hypnosis bear a considerable relationship to their own hypnotic performance. This relationship could hardly obtain unless two hypotheses were correct: first . . . that 'when

---

be". Characteristic kinds of responses are given by individuals, according to their personality structures.

[12] In this test, the subject is shown a series of pictures and asked to "make up a story" about them. During the course of this procedure, the subject reveals his fantasies (conscious and unconscious), usually without becoming aware that he is doing so. One such picture shows what appears to be one man trying to hypnotize another.

someone attempts to interpret a complex social situation he is apt to tell as much about himself as he is about the phenomena on which attention is focused,' for which reason the Thematic Apperception Test 'is an effective means of disclosing a subject's regnant preoccupations and some of the unconscious trends which underlie them'; second, that what the subject tells about himself in this way, in other words, the attitude which he reveals, is a genuine determination of his responsiveness in the hypnotic test."

It would be our supposition that if a subject's responses to the hypnosis picture did indeed disclose some of the significant "unconscious trends", and if our knowledge were more complete regarding the specific "unconscious trends" which are related to hypnotizability, this correlation would be significantly higher. Although this statement may appear to be self-evident, it is made in order to call attention to the fact that the above described approach, while it is the most promising to date, is limited by the fact that it elicits data from a level that seems closer to conscious attitudes than to "unconscious trends". It might be that on the basis of stories given in response to pictures unrelated to hypnosis deeper and more significant attitudes might be elicited.

White has tried to isolate some of the "deeper" factors crucial for hypnotizability. He has formulated his hypothesis in the vocabulary worked out by Murray and his associates in their cooperative study at the Harvard Psychological Clinic (103). He concludes that "the attraction of passivity is of central importance in determining the outcome of an hypnotic experiment with those subjects who are not fundamentally unwilling."[13] He adds, however, that in the deeply hypnotizable subjects, one finds those who respond in a drowsy, sluggish way and those who are alert and obedient. Only the former are really maximal in the variables that indicate "passivity"; the latter are about average on "passivity" but show a great need for "deference" and receive uniformly low ratings on

[13] p. 460.

48   HYPNOTHERAPY: A SURVEY OF THE LITERATURE

the need for "autonomy". These results suggest that a person
may enter into the hypnotic relationship "on the strength
of two quite different motives".

Rosenzweig's "triadic hypothesis" (105) has been developed
along similar lines in that he, too, employs an experimental
rather than a clinical approach and in that his formulations
are conceived largely in terms of the Murray concepts although
he uses psychoanalytic vocabulary as well. He has employed
the correlational and the Thematic Apperception approaches
in collaboration with Sarason. He states the "triadic hypothesis"
as follows: "Hypnotizability as a personality trait is to be found
in positive association with repression as a preferred mechanism
of defense and with impunitiveness as a characteristic type
of immediate reaction to frustration."[14] On the basis of correlation coefficients obtained from measures of reaction to
frustration, liability to the repression of unpleasant experiences,
and hypnotizability "or suggestibility", he concludes that the
"components of the triadic hypothesis" are positively associated
(105).[15] He adds: "It was found reciprocally that those individuals who do not utilize repression as a mechanism of defense
are characteristically extrapunitive and nonhypnotizable." From
the Thematic Apperception approach the authors conclude:

> "The experimenter and an independent judge were
> able to differentiate hypnotizable from nonhypnotiz-
> able individuals on the basis of the response to an
> 'hypnosis' picture to a statistically significant degree.
> The characteristics of the verbal and adverbial phrases
> employed by the nonhypnotizable subject were typi-
> cally extrapunitive in their expression of fear, aggres-
> sion, and suspicion. Those of the hypnotizable
> individual were typically impunitive in conveying
> cooperativeness, conciliation, and acceptance of the

[14]The term "impunitiveness" refers here to that characteristic of a person that
leads him to react in a frustrating situation by glossing over or rationalizing
rather than with externally directed (extrapunitive) or internally directed (in-
trapunitive) aggression.

[15] p. 19.

presence and success of hypnosis. An analysis of the stories in terms of needs reveals deference, affiliation, and abasement to be characteristic of the hypnotizable subjects, and autonomy and anxiety of the non-hypnotizable."[16]

They state that, although both the quantitative and qualitative approaches offer confirmatory evidence for the "triadic hypothesis", further study is indicated.

It must be apparent even from this brief survey of the meagre literature that there is neither clinical nor experimental data sufficient to draw any conclusions regarding either the personality characteristics of the good hypnotic subject or the psychiatric syndromes that are most susceptible to hypnosis. There exist reports of successful hypnosis in almost every nosological category and there also are reports of utter failure in all.

Although we do not know what makes an individual susceptible to hypnosis, we do know that such susceptibility is not a static property of the person which consistently appears under any and all conditions. The therapist must be constantly aware of the need to alter the "psychological atmosphere" in line with the *immediate* emotional needs of the patient which seem to influence susceptibility. If the patient is frightened or consciously over-anxious to please, he will be a more difficult subject. Often, a skillful therapist may neutralize such obstacles by deferring his attempts until he has explored what Fisher (94) has called "the areas of anxiety". Curiously enough, "faith" or lack of it seems to make no difference whatever. Forel (96) has pointed out that many patients who deride hypnosis are often markedly susceptible whereas many who "believe" remain entirely refractory. This observation is confirmed by the present reviewers' experience.

It is a curious fact that a patient who is refractory during the first two or three trials may go into deep hypnosis during the fourth attempt. Tuckey (108) would usually stop after the

[16] p. 165.

fourth or fifth unsuccessful session. On the other hand, Moll (101) has sometimes succeeded only after forty sittings and Vogt (109) tried seven-hundred times fruitlessly to obtain somnambulism and succeeded on the seven-hundred and first attempt. Most hypnotherapists do not persevere or find it expedient to invest time much beyond Tuckey's limits. We offer these figures only to suggest that susceptibility to hypnosis seems to be a fairly fluid characteristic of the person which, if latent, may be brought out under conditions which are, for him, psychologically optimal.

CHAPTER FOUR

THERAPEUTIC APPLICATIONS

The need for a review of the specific applications of hypnosis in psychotherapy is immediately evident to anyone who makes the most cursory survey of discussions of hypnotherapy in current textbooks of psychiatry. For the most part, with the notable exception of Kraines (178) the authors present this form of treatment as if its history had stopped sixty-five years ago with the early editions of Bernheim's *Suggestive Therapeutics* (119). Only the most primitive form of hypnotherapy (namely, the removal of symptoms by direct suggestion) is mentioned and even this is usually presented in a way that hopelessly confuses even this form of treatment with the deceptions and sadistic trickeries of faradic brushes and the like.

Actually there has taken place a considerable development since the "classical period" of hypnosis and it is our purpose in this chapter to present a review of the varieties of hypnotherapy that are being used currently. We shall summarize the methods, their advantages and limitations, and the kinds of cases treated by each.

There are at least six different ways described in the literature in which hypnosis may be applied therapeutically: 1. Prolonged hypnosis without direct suggestion or exploration. 2. Direct suggestion of symptom-disappearance. 3. Direct suggestion of disappearance of attitudes underlying symptoms. 4. Abreaction of traumatic experience. 5. The use of specialized hypnotic techniques. 6. Hypnoanalysis.

1. *Prolonged Hypnosis.*

This method has been used most extensively by Wetter-strand (242). The patient is hypnotized as deeply as possible and is allowed to remain in hypnosis for an extended period, much as in prolonged narcosis or "Dauerschlaf". Depending on its initial depth, the hypnotic state may or may not have to be supported by small drug dosages. Wetterstrand, who frequently kept his patients in a deep hypnosis for periods of several days, likened the therapeutic effect of this to the healing power of deep sleep. During this period, no direct therapeutic suggestions are given and no explorations made. Schilder and Kauders (219) who have used a modification of this technique say: "We believe that, in addition to the physical effect of the sleep, the psychic elaboration which the person devotes during sleep, to his experience, also has value."[17] They report especially good results in the treatment of stubborn tics and in acute conversion symptoms (e. g., psychogenic vomiting). Rothenberg (216) has had similar success with such symptoms.

This technique is not widely used because of the practical difficulties involved. It may be applied successfully in a hospital situation where adequate nursing care is available.

2. *Direct Suggestion of Symptom-disappearance.*

This is the oldest and still most widely used of the techniques of hypnotherapy. Hypnosis is induced by one of the methods described in Chapter Two and direct suggestions are made to the patient that his symptoms will disappear. The prototype for this primitive, though often effective, technique is Bernheim's description of his own approach:

> "For example, a child is brought to me with a pain like muscular rheumatism in its arm dating back four or five days; the arm is painful to pressure; the child cannot lift it to its head. I say to him, 'Shut your eyes, my child, and go to sleep.' I hold his eyelids

[17] p. 97.

closed and go on talking to him. 'You are asleep and you will keep on sleeping until I tell you to wake up. You are sleeping very well, as if you were in your bed; you are perfectly well and comfortable; your arms and legs and your whole body are asleep and you cannot move.' I take my fingers off his eyelids and they remain closed; I put his arms up, and they remain so. Then, touching the painful arm, I say, 'The pain has gone away. You have no more pain anywhere; you can move your arm without any pain; and when you wake up you will not feel any more pain. It will not come back any more.' In order to increase the force of the suggestion by embodying it, so to speak, in a material sensation, following M. Liebeault's example, I suggest a feeling of warmth *loco dolenti*. The heat takes the place of the pain. I say to the child, 'You feel that your arm is warm; the warmth increases, and you have no more pain.' "[18]

This is the simplest therapeutic application of hypnosis and the one that most closely resembles the magical or the miraculous. The literature published between 1880 and 1900 is replete with case reports both of temporary relief and of some follow-up studies where this relief has been maintained. Although there have been reports of frequent relapses or formation of substitute-symptoms after a "successful" removal of symptoms, there exist many instances of permanent cure as well.

Janet (172) reported a fair number of permanent cures particularly when the disturbance was treated shortly after its inception. Hollander (167) has pointed out also that, in his experience, relapses may be averted by avoiding mechanical suggestions that are not adapted to the patient. He says that relapses are not more frequent in hypnotherapy than they are in any other form of treatment and that no other psychotherapy can claim so many rapid and lasting cures.

More recently Wells (242) has added to the record a striking and detailed account of permanent cure by direct suggestion.

[18] pp. 207-8.

This was the case of a young college student who had suffered a constant disabling headache for five years after suffering a trauma to one of his eyes. He had consulted several internists, and had been placed on a strict regime of diet and bowel control by a neurologist. These measures had been completely without result. During this period, he had showed also almost all of the major symptoms of hysteria (hysterical contractures, fugues, nocturnal somnambulism, amnesia). Here, as is so often the case in the method of direct suggestion, the technique was almost absurdly simple. Wells (242) describes it as follows: " 'When I count up to ten your headache will entirely disappear.' I counted up to ten and Mr. Jones reported that his headache had stopped. I then said, 'When I count from ten to twenty the headache will be gone permanently.' Then I counted from ten to twenty. I explained to Mr. Jones, while he was still in deep hypnosis, that the evidence was clear that the headache had been purely hallucinatory and that no ill effects could follow its complete eradication by hypnotic methods. I stated that when he came out of hypnosis he would find himself permanently freed from the pain, and that he would have complete amnesia for all that had occurred during the entire hypnotic period." For the first time in four years, the patient was able to sleep normally and the "strained facial expression of pain" had disappeared. The fugue states were now explored by breaking through the amnesia in deep hypnosis and have not since recurred.

There is scarcely any functional disturbance that has not been successfully treated by the technique of direct suggestion in hypnosis. To attempt a compilation of "types of cases treated by this method" becomes an almost impossible and even pointless task. Individual therapists offer in their summaries long lists of the ailments they have treated with this approach; the scientific value of these lists is limited by the fact that there is little or no agreement among them (222). Thus, for example, Forel (153) has enthusiastically maintained his particularly good therapeutic results with cases of all kinds of addiction:

alcoholism, morphinism, and so forth. Wetterstrand (243) has reported good success with these cases, with only three recidivists out of forty cases of morphine addiction. Heyer (164) has supported these data. Tuckey (241), on the other hand, believes from his experience that the majority of addicts treated by direct suggestion soon suffer a relapse. Schilder and Kauders (219) also report negative results on the hypnotherapy of addicts.

Almost every syndrome which we might now label "psychosomatic" has been reported successfully treated by direct suggestion. Warts have been removed (121), all varieties of menstrual disturbance have been treated (153) (179), and skin diseases like psoriasis (245) are included in the list, as are asthma (155) (233), muscular rheumatism (246), migraine (239), constipation (153), epilepsy (166), sea-sickness (165) and insomnia (241). We present this sampling only to suggest the unlimited scope given this method, particularly during what Janet (172) has facetiously labelled the "palmy days of hypnosis". The *Zeitschrift für Hypnotismus* includes scores of reports of this sort (138). A typical article of this kind is Bauer's paper (116) on a group of patients treated during a single summer at Forel's polyclinic. Even symptoms of known organic origin have been alleviated by direct suggestion. Reinhold's results with postencephalitic Parkinsonism lead Schilder and Kauders (219) to the statement that: "At any rate, these observations at least suggest that even organic symptoms may be influenced in hypnosis, and that the accessibility to influence in hypnosis may not always be made use of in setting up a differential diagnosis between a functional and an organic disturbance."[19]

In addition, all known psychological aberrations are to be found in a compilation of cases treated by direct suggestion. Although most authors agree that obsessions and compulsions are particularly unresponsive to this technique (173), there are reports of the successful treatment even of these (244)

[19] p. 112.

(137), especially if they are mild or of recent origin (164) (219). There seems to be a fairly good agreement that if a hysterical patient is hypnotizable in the first place, he is "one of the most grateful objects of hypnotherapy" (219). Janet (172) says that in his breakdown of cases, the paraplegias, mutisms, amauroses, contractures, sleep-walking, and so forth, are those that show the greatest reliability and permanence of cure when treated by this method. This does not mean, however, that hysterics are regularly amenable to this form of treatment because there is much evidence, as we shall see, that hysterics are frequently refractory to all attempts to hypnotize them. Heyer (164), on the other hand, warns against the use of hypnosis in "grave" hysteria, saying that severe hysterical attacks may occur and one may lose rapport with the subject. The possibility of an "attack" may actually be utilized, however, as a therapeutic lever, as will be shown in the later discussions.

Phobias are generally not regarded as suitable for treatment by direct suggestion (248) although here again there are reports of their successful hypnotherapeutic treatment (219).

Speech disturbances have frequently been cured by direct suggestion (166) (181), although recent trends in treatment have been away from a simple statement that the difficulty would disappear and more toward a manipulation of underlying attitudes.

We have by no means exhausted the list of types of disorders treated by direct suggestion nor have we attempted to include even a fraction of the papers presenting these results. Tuckey (241), whose book on direct suggestion is perhaps the best of its kind, has said: " . . . whenever we find a chronic disease resisting the usual methods of treatment, suggestion may be thought of as a useful ally." In the recent literature, the only two kinds of cases where this method is generally regarded as of no value are the psychoses and "true melancholia". In the latter it is usually contraindicated (219). Heyer (164) has felt it is not advisable in schizophrenia because it may become pathologically elaborated.

Direct suggestion was used far more extensively with psychiatric casualties in World War I than in World War II. *The Lancet* and the *Journal of the Royal Army Medical Corps* contained, particularly in the early days of the war, numerous articles describing the use of this technique in the war neuroses. Hurst (168), who was at first one of the best known advocates of this method, later felt it important to enlist the active participation of the soldier in his treatment and to combine "persuasion and education" with hypnosis, with the emphasis distinctly on the former. Tombleson (238) in 1917 registered a plea for the use of direct suggestion in his description of twenty cases treated by "hypnotic suggestion". He describes the rapid cure of many cases of "neurasthenia" and "psychasthenia" (which, from his description, sound more like cases of conversion hysteria) and even of hyperthyroidism in soldiers.

Trotter (240) writing in 1918, following the early work of Hurst, described a treatment for what he called the "motor psychoneuroses" among war casualties. Although he does not label it as hypnotherapy, his description makes it quite clear that essentially the same principles are involved. He, too, felt the necessity for supplementing direct suggestion with "persuasion" and "explanation".

The reaction against methods that sought merely rapid symptom-relief became increasingly evident during this period. Thus, even Ross (213) writing in *The Lancet* in 1918 comments ironically on the use of "electricity, hypnotism and manipulation". Here, as is so frequently the case, he confuses the use of sadistic deception and terror typified in Yealland's (247) treatment of conversion hysteria by faradism with direct suggestion in hypnosis.

There was fairly unanimous agreement, however, that in the recovery of amnesic periods, hypnosis was of great value in the war situation (196), although here too the fact of its being an auxiliary technique, and not the core of the psychotherapy of amnesias, was emphasized by McDougall (187) and others.

In World War II, hypnotherapy of any sort was not widely employed. There are few reports of the use of direct suggestion of the classical type. Modified techniques applied in a context of substantial psychotherapeutic "tact" have been used by a few physicians. Fisher (152) has reported on his findings with several hypnotherapeutic techniques, direct suggestion having been one among them. He achieved one of his most striking successes by using this method to cure hyperhydrosis and painful calluses in a coast guardsman. Although he regards this as simply a "symptomatic cure", he emphasizes the importance of such cures if they are instituted early. Miller (191) and Kardiner (174) recommended the use of hypnotherapy in the war neuroses also.

Before proceeding to a description of the modified methods of direct suggestion in hypnosis, we shall summarize the values and limitations of the method of simply suggesting symptom-disappearance. If the patient responds at all to this kind of treatment, this response is usually fairly prompt and the improvement rapid. Very little specialized training or experience in the specific techniques of psychotherapy is necessary in order to achieve good therapeutic results with this approach, inasmuch as no attempt is made to "uncover" the root of the difficulty. Training and experience in the technique of hypnosis are the only prerequisites. The therapeutic leverage consists largely of whatever deep unconscious needs are stirred in the patient in his relationship to the therapist during the hypnosis. We do not understand the nature of this relationship, but this does not alter the fact that by dint of its existence, the patient may obtain relief from his symptoms, sometimes temporarily and often permanently.

On the other hand, in the advantages of this method lie also its limitations. Because it is, in effect, an attempt to suppress the patient's symptoms, it is not possible for the patient to gain any insight into the emotional roots of his difficulty. Accordingly (and this is especially true in disturbances that have remained untreated for any length of time), the possibility of relapse or of the formation of a substitute symptom is always present, although not inevitable. Another limitation of this method is that it usually requires a fairly deep hypnosis for rapid results, although there have been reports of successful symptom-removal even in light states of hypnosis (153) (223) or in what Sidis called "hypnoid states".

3. Direct Suggestion of Disappearance of Attitudes Underlying Symptoms.

The work of Bernheim has been cited as typical of the approach that commands symptom-disappearance, but a close study of his writings reveals that he himself went beyond this in his clinical work. Although most of his followers directed their attention largely to the direct suppression of symptoms, Bernheim shows himself to be a more imaginative therapist by the following:

> "The mode of suggestion should also be varied and adapted to the special suggestibility of the subject. A simple word does not always suffice in impressing the idea upon the mind. It is sometimes necessary to reason, to prove, to convince; in some cases, to affirm decidedly; in others, to insinuate gently; for in the condition of sleep just as in the waking condition the moral individuality of each subject persists according to his character, his inclinations, his special impressionability, and so forth. Hypnosis does not run all its subjects into a uniform mould, and make pure and simple automatons out of them, moved solely by the will of the magnetizer."[20]

The flexibility of method was taken up with enthusiasm and developed by those workers who were embarrassed by the complete absence of rational psychotherapeutics in classical hypnotherapy. We have discussed the dissatisfaction of

[20] p. 210.

several investigators with the comparatively shallow technique of direct suggestion and mentioned their introduction of "persuasion and re-education". It is as if this variant of hypnotherapy represents an historical compromise between the "irrational" appeal of hypnosis with the "rational" appeal of a naive common-sense psychotherapy. Its adherents represent a mediating position between the classical hypnotists and the almost moralistic approach of a man like Du Bois, who denounced hypnosis, saying it brought "a blush to my cheek".

This trend first found articulate expression in the early decades of this century in the work of Prince, Coriat, Sidis, and others. A typical example is an article written in 1907 by Prince and Coriat entitled, "Cases Illustrating the Educational Treatment of the Psychoneuroses" (210). Although there are, even in this article, case records of cure by direct symptom suppression, and by indirect suggestion (fictitious "magnets"), emphasis is laid on re-education. In one typical account, the authors describe their treatment of "psycho-epileptic attacks simulating Jacksonian epilepsy". In hypnosis, the patient recalled that an earlier fright had produced in her what she called a "delirium" and that people around had then remarked that apparently, like her mother, she had epilepsy. The treatment then consisted of telling her while she was in deep hypnosis that she did not have epilepsy, but that she did have an unfounded fear. Thus, the fear would disappear and along with it, the epileptic attacks. The patient was told that now she "realized and believed". The attacks ceased immediately.

Although one is struck by the naiveté of this psychotherapy, one cannot but be impressed at the same time with the records of clinical results. Here, as in the use of direct suggestion, it would appear that on the basis of the relationship with the therapist (and whatever else being in hypnosis consists of), the patient is able to give up symptoms with only a meagre and rudimentary insight into their origin. We have seen both from the results of "direct suggestion" and from "faith-cures" that symptoms are relinquished even in the complete absence of insight. The importance, therefore, of the introduction of even so primitive a variety of insight lies in its attempt to bolster the patient against future attacks.

Similar lines were followed by Sidis (224) and Donley (139) for some cases. For instance, an obsessional neurosis in a twenty-one-year-old student was "cured" within less than three weeks. The young man had the insistent thought after reading a newspaper article that a comet might strike the earth and destroy it. At first he had attempted to deal with this idea by making elaborate mathematical calculations to prove to himself the statistical remoteness of this possibility. This was futile. When he applied for help to Donley, he was put into the hypnoidal state and asked to recall when he had first had this idea. It is uncertain just what Donley did at this point. He says:

> "Having completed his narrative he was then given an explanation of the origin, the nature and the significance of his ideas. In view of his superior intelligence he was able to comprehend what was said to him with apparently little difficulty. He declared himself after half an hour's treatment to feel much relieved mentally and less disturbed physically, in the sense that he felt less of the nervous bodily trembling of which he complained."

He was given another treatment a week later and ten days after this he announced himself as being practically over his fear and had since had no recurrence of this idea.

One could continue indefinitely to add illustrations of this general approach. The extreme to which the "rational" approach was pushed is shown in Brown's (127) "golden rule of psychotherapy": the therapist must never become angry and he must never permit the patient to become angry. The cool and reasonable character of the psychotherapy would be interfered with if such emotional expression were admitted. In this connection an earlier paper by Van Renterghen (211) is of interest. In treating a case of torticollis by hypnosis, he emphasized at the same time that the patient control his anger during the course of treatment which lasted several months. The patient was cured and told van Renterghen, "You treated me not only for my spasms but for my rages."

The historical significance of the "rational" approach in hypnotherapy lies in the fact that this trend reflected the growing awareness of the importance of giving the patient some understanding of his difficulty. That it took so intellectualized a form is ascribable to the fact that during the first decades of this century the laws governing unconscious processes were as yet little accepted.

During the period between 1900 and 1920, men like Hollander (166) (167), Miller (192), and Gerrish (155) supported this point of view. More recently Kraines (178) summarizes this method as follows:

> "In the therapeutic suggestions, it is not only important to suggest that the symptoms clear up, but to suggest that the basic emotional difficulties be dealt with in a more hygienic manner. Indeed, far more emphasis should be placed on the underlying factors than on the symptom. This line of suggestion presupposes that the patient was examined and studied before the hypnotic treatment was begun and that an analysis was made of the etiologic factors. Hypnosis thus becomes a valuable aid in enabling the patient to carry out the retraining of the personality, as well as 'suggesting away the symptom'."

Illustrating this technique he gives a fragment of the hypnotherapy of a case of torticollis:

> "Now relax your neck; relax it still more. Your head feels so very good, and all the tension is gone. It relaxes still more and still more. Now the head begins to straighen itself out. It turns to the midline— and your head tips to the opposite side. Good. Now your chin is down and your head is in normal position. It will continue to be normal. It feels so good now. Your head will remain normal. (After these

specific suggestions, the emotional bases behind the symptom should be dealt with.) Your aversion to your employer will disappear, and you'll regard him as an old and disagreeable person; but you will not be affected by his manners. You will not be disturbed by your husband's irritability but will just let his anger fall off you—like water off a duck's back. You will learn not to let anything bother you. That's why you will face everything straightforwardly. Your head is straight now and will stay that way. Next time you come here you will go to sleep more easily and quickly, and until then your head will remain in midline. Now gradually wake up, and you feel very well. Wake up completely."

It is quite obvious from this account that Kraines had concluded from his preliminary examination that the torticollis symptom was a symbolic representation of the patient's reluctance to "face things straightforwardly" and thus directed his suggestions both at the symptom itself and at its underlying "meaning".

Recently, the applications of hypnotherapy to speech disorders have followed this approach (185) (181). Usually, direct suggestions of confidence, ease, relaxation, are given rather than suggestions that the stuttering or stammering will disappear.

The choice of which "underlying attitudes" to attack depends largely on the preconceptions of the individual therapist regarding the essential nature of emotional illness. Thus, the conclusions regarding the etiology may be formulated at many different "psychic levels". Morgan (195) in 1924 elicited from a previously inaccessible suicidal girl the fact that she feared she was pregnant, and that she had been taught that "sex is wrong"; he met this therapeutically by telling the patient that sex is not wrong and that it is the task of a normal woman to recognize her womanhood and to finally marry the man of her choice. Although he calls this "a direct psychoanalytic statement", it will be at once apparent to anyone familiar with psychoanalytic theory or technique that this is an extremely crude derivative. The patient responded very well, however, and after three hypnotic sessions began to recover from what had "looked like a case of hebephrenic dementia praecox".

The recent work of Muniz (199) (200) (201) (202) has been along similar lines. Although he, too, speaks of the combined use of "psychoanalysis and hypnotism", he makes psychodynamic deductions of a shallow variety and then uses these in formulating direct suggestions to the patient. In one case of "anxiety neurosis" he attempted at first to treat the patient by a reorganization of her routine and by giving her medication. When, after several months, no real progress had taken place, he hypnotized her and utilized his insight into the fact that she had first developed symptoms when her servant had fallen ill and she had been torn between a desire to help her servant and a desire to flee the entire situation. The superficiality of this "analysis" is at once evident. Despite this limitation, the patient began to improve rapidly under the newly instituted treatment and has remained well.

This is an instructive "natural experiment" because it suggests that the normal, everyday relationship of this patient with Muniz, who was her family physician, did not provide sufficient therapeutic leverage nor did the indirect suggestion of regimen-change or medication. Apparently, the hypnotic relationship did introduce a significantly new and important element to make the difference. Here, as in all clinical reports, one cannot be certain of the precise factors that are directly responsible for the cure. One can rely only on the faithfulness of the therapist's report. Schilder (218) brought this technique of hypnotherapy more definitely within the frame of psychoanalytic theory. He compared it with the similar technique of direct suggestion of symptom-disappearance as follows:

> "We have described the method of hypnosis used as direct suggestion. The suggestion can be directed against the symptom as such. In some cases it can-

not be avoided; for instance, in tics and in organ neuroses, where the genesis of the symptom is not ascertained. Direct suggestion can also be used in clearly formulating the problems to the patient and suggesting to him that on the basis of the insight, symptoms will disappear. This method is preferable; and it is, of course, necessary in order to formulate the suggestion properly that one knows something about the genesis of the symptoms. Preliminary work in this respect will be necessary. One should be careful in suggesting problems and their solutions, unless one has a sufficient insight oneself. . . . The full implications of hypnosis can only be understood in connection with the general conduct of a psychotherapy. The relation of the patient to the physician has to be fully understood if one wants to make the correct use of hypnosis as a therapeutic method. In the limits discussed above, hypnosis can be of help in short psychotherapy."

A list of comparable length and variety to that described in connection with simple direct suggestion could be compiled for the method described above. Here, too, all of the usual psychiatric syndromes, with the exception of the psychoses (in the modern sense) have been treated with success by some therapists. However, this method of hypnotherapy has been somewhat more limited in its scope of cases[21] and has been used more frequently for the symptoms of conversion hysteria than for anything else. For example Schilder and Kauders (219) say:

"We recently treated a young man who always failed at examinations owing to a feeling of acute fear

[21] Janet (172) points out that there was literally no illness, functional or organic, which was not treated by the early mesmerists and that in fact Liébeault had treated all sorts of disorders regarded as strictly organic (as an antidote to poison, for anemia, pulmonary tuberculosis, migraine, and so forth.) It is probably not an accident that those forms of therapy that seem to rest on a concrete or symbolic relationship with a parent-surrogate also do not restrict themselves in their scope (Christian Science, "miracle-cures", and the like). It is as if a belief in omnipotence is revived and thus "anything is possible". This belief is sometimes rewarded by the cure of a psychosomatic disturbance where irreversible organic changes have not yet taken place.

and terror. It turned out that whenever he was present at an examination, he experienced a revival of his fear of his over-severe father. The suggestion was therefore aimed not only against his fear of examinations, but also against his attitude of terror toward his father. It is therefore our effort always to get down to the psychic causes and to combat these psychic causes by means of suggestion. But it is evident at once that such a treatment absolutely requires an intimate association with the patient. We are of a view that such intimate association with the patient will be more fruitful if the physician has a knowledge of psychoanalysis and is capable of applying the psychoanalytic technique in the conversations preceding the hypnosis."

We fully agree that a technique that attempts to go beyond the treatment of symptoms requires far more specialized training in psychotherapy than the method of direct suggestion. This, from the point of view of ready and wide applicability, is its disadvantage. However, insofar as such a technique provides the patient with some understanding of his problem, it is a more reliable and substantial method of hypnotherapy. It may take somewhat longer than a course of treatment by direct suggestion, particularly if a systematic attempt is made to establish the specific etiological factors underlying the symptom before the suggestion is formulated.

4. Abreaction of Traumatic Experiences.

Although the concept of "catharsis" was used by Aristotle in connection with the release of pent-up emotion (as in aesthetic experience), its introduction into the history of psychotherapy generally and of hypnotherapy in particular is fairly recent. The third and final edition (1930) of Bramwell's five-hundred page textbook on hypnosis (122) does not include either the term "abreaction" or "catharsis" in its index. It is actually difficult to explain such an oversight inasmuch as Breuer and Freud (125) had used the term "abreaction" in connection with the re-living of repressed affect thirty-five years earlier.

Schilder (218) gives Janet credit for first having employed in his therapeutic approach the technique of searching for affect-charged traumatic memories. He admits that Breuer had had an accidental earlier experience with "abreaction" when a patient developed a spontaneous hypnosis but says that Janet's publications (170) preceded Breuer's. Janet himself has argued his priority with some bitterness in several places (171) (172).

Janet (172) gives many interesting case reports to illustrate this method. A well-known example is that of "Marie", a girl of nineteen who suffered every month from convulsions, delirium, and fits of shivering accompanying her menstruation. She had other hysterical symptoms as well: an anesthesia of the left side of the face and amaurosis of the left eye. In hypnosis, Marie recovered with much emotion her terror at menstruating at the age of thirteen, and her frantic efforts to check the flow by getting into a tub of cold water, shivering and trembling all the while. She recalled also a "terrible fright" in this connection, when she had seen an old woman fall and cover the stairs with blood. Other memories related to the anesthesia were recovered also. None of these was accessible to her normal waking consciousness. Following the recovery of these memories, Marie's "hysterical crises" ceased. We shall defer the theoretical discussion of the mechanism of "abreaction" until we have concluded a full presentation of the method.

Freud in his *Autobiography* (154) describes Breuer's first experience with the cathartic method as follows:

> "When Breuer took over her case it presented a variegated picture of paralyses with contractures, inhibitions and states of mental confusion. A chance observation showed her physician that she could be relieved of these clouded states of consciousness if she were induced to express in words the affective phantasy by which she was at the moment dominated. From this discovery, Breuer arrived at a new method of treatment. He put her into a deep hypnosis and made her

tell him each time what it was that was oppressing her mind. In her waking state the girl could no more describe than other patients how her symptoms had arisen, and she could discover no link between them and any experiences of her life. In hypnosis she immediately revealed the missing connection. It turned out that all her symptoms went back to moving events which she had experienced while nursing her father; that is to say, her symptoms had a meaning and were residues or reminiscences of those emotional situations. It turned out in most instances that there had been some thought or impulse which she had had to suppress while she was by her father's sick-bed, and that, in place of it, as a substitute for it, the symptom had afterwards appeared. But as a rule the symptom was not the precipitate of a single such 'traumatic' scene, but the result of a summation of a number of situations. When the patient recalled a situation of this kind in a hallucinatory way under hypnosis and carried through to its conclusion, with a free expression of emotion, the mental act which she had originally suppressed, the symptom was abolished and did not return. By this procedure, Breuer succeeded, after long and painful efforts, in relieving his patient of all her symptoms."[22]

It appears that the recovery of the significant traumatic experiences with the attendant emotion may take place at any point on a scale of emotional intensity. The patient may recall the previously inaccessible memory with the accompanying statement, "I feel now much as I did then," a kind of muted echo of the original feeling with a complete awareness of current reality or, at the other extreme, he may actually appear to be re-living the episode in an uninhibited and overtly tempestuous manner, screaming, wailing, cowering or trembling.

The "abreactive" method was taken up with much enthusiasm by many who had been dissatisfied with the technique of direct suggestion, which provided neither the therapist nor the patient with any understanding of the etiology of the ill-

[22] pp. 33-35.

ness. This kind of treatment was actively investigated in the first decades of this century by many workers, among them Sidis (223) (224), Donley (139), Goldwyn (157), Taplin (233), Loewenfeld (186), Prince (209), William Brown (130) (131), McDougall (188), and Hadfield (161). For the most part, this work was essentially like that of Janet, Freud, and Breuer, although the attempts to "re-associate" or "synthesize" the recovered memory with the normal ego of the person vary from a dependence on the mere ventilation of the traumatic event to a systematic effort to re-integrate the newly discovered material with the current life of the patient.[23]

This method has been employed with a more restricted group of disease-entities than either of the two methods previously discussed. Most of the work conducted by Janet, Freud, and Breuer was with hysterical patients. Freud (125) says, however:

> "Yet, it sometimes happened that in spite of the diagnosis of hysteria, the therapeutic results were very poor, and even the analysis revealed nothing of importance. At other times I attempted to treat cases by Breuer's method, which no one took for hysteria, and I found that I could influence them, and even cure them. Such, for example, was my experience with obsessions, the real obsessions of Westphal's type, in cases which did not show a single feature of hysteria."[24]

Goldwyn (157) and Donley (139) support Freud in this finding, both having worked successfully with a number of obsessional neuroses. Hadfield (159) (161) reports the best

---

[23] Although Hadfield and later Taylor referred to their therapeutic applications of hypnosis as "hypno-analysis" and Brown speaks of "hypnotic analysis", we include these men in this section because their techniques seem closer to the classical use of "abreaction" than to recent methods of hypnotherapy which attempt to combine hypnosis with the specific techniques of psychodynamic psychotherapy and of psychoanalysis. We shall discuss the latter in the section on "hypnoanalysis".

[24] pp. 198-199.

results of this method with "motor symptoms", especially paralyses, and with "sensory disturbances" which remain after an organic illness (with which the pain was originally associated) has been cured. Taylor (234) has also reported success with motor symptoms, and Connellan (135) with depressions. Copeland and Kitching (137) have attempted to use this approach with alcoholics but have thus far been able to report only temporary cures. Phobias have been in a few instances successfully treated by this technique: Smith (228) has recently reported the cure of a nineteen-year-old youth who suffered from an intense fear of the dark. The most striking aspect of his report is the fact that he was able to recover verifiable memories of the original traumatic episode which took place, apparently, before the boy was yet three years old.

There is general agreement that, if the patient is hypnotizable, the cathartic method is the method of choice in cases of amnesia (213). Schilder (218) has said that he has had success with this approach almost exclusively with amnesias and allied states, and has been disappointed in his attempts to treat other functional disorders.

"Abreaction" has been found particularly suitable to that group of psychological disturbances lately called the "traumatic neuroses of war". Hadfield (159) (161) has reported on his treatment of between six and seven hundred cases in the period from 1915 to 1920, psychiatric casualties of World War I. He describes it as follows:

> "The patient, hypnotized, is told that when the physician puts his hand on his forehead he will feel himself back in the trenches, or under fire; that he will visualize all the circumstances when he was blown up or buried, and live again through all the emotional experiences concerned. He is encouraged to describe them as he experiences them. The patient usually becomes disoriented, shows signs of great emotion, trembles, perspires, engages in violent movements, and may be speechless with horror or cry out with fear."

He warns that the immediate effect of recalling the traumatic experience may be an exacerbation of the symptom or the appearance of substitute-symptoms: "The headache disappears but gives place to acute anxiety; or in addition to the pain in the back, the patient begins to vomit." He may have the typical repetitive battle-dream and be more disturbed temporarily than he was before the inception of treatment. He says no harm is done if direct suggestions are given to alleviate the acute attack, providing this is then followed by further exploration and what Hadfield terms "readjustment". This is constituted by a repeated "working through" of the experience until the patient can actually accept the fact that the original trauma is no longer a threat to him. He says that he has usually obtained satisfactory results within twelve to fifteen sessions.

William Brown was one of the most enthusiastic exponents of the cathartic method during World War I. He restricted this form of psychotherapy largely to those soldiers showing major hysterical symptoms and says that in every one of 121 cases of hysterical mutism this method restored the power of speech in a few minutes (128) (129). He describes a typical treatment of a case of "shell-shock" as follows:

> "It is the case of a gunner who was admitted to the hospital where I was working, after he had spent two years in military hospitals of different kinds. He was suffering from a tremor of the right hand, dating from the time when he had been blown up at Ypres. He did not remember anything more until he reached his first hospital, and the memory of this interval had never been recalled to him by any of the doctors he had previously seen. I sent him to sleep—that took just about three seconds—and then suggested to him that he should live again through the experience of Ypres. He did so, and began to shout out all sorts of things which showed what had been happening at the time. German shells were falling nearer and nearer the gun pit. He was apparently serving the gun, and someone else was handing him the ammunition, and this person had evidently lost his head, for my patient

shouted out: 'What the — do you mean by pulling
the — pin out of that — fuse?' Then I noticed that he
was going through the pantomime of moving the
handle (to serve the gun) with his right hand; his
hand began to shake violently and soon he was shaking all over, but especially in his right hand. Then he
suddenly became absolutely still. I suggested to him
that he would continue to remember all that he had
just gone through and then woke him up. He looked
at his hand, which was then absolutely still, with
amazement and expressed his gratitude, but his mind
still appeared somewhat confused, so I told him to go
off and sleep it off. An hour later he came back and
told me that he had not been to sleep, but that he had
been thinking it all over. He knew everything that had
happened, and told me that he had not been suffering
from shell-shock, but gun-shock. His gun had been
blown up, and the emotion which this experience ex-
cited in him had been bottled up for two years, with
the result that he suffered from this tremor of the
hand. The next morning he was able to shave himself
with an ordinary razor, for the first time since his
illness."

In his report on the treatment of "shell-shock" at an advanced neurological center, he concludes that whereas "mental
analysis" (employing the technique of free association) is the
ideal method, abreactive hypnotherapy is an "aid" and a
"short-cut". Similar results are reported by Taylor (234) and
Ross (214).

Although the "abreactive method" has been used extensively
in World War II, the alteration in consciousness which is necessary for such a "re-living" has usually been brought about by
drugs rather than by the verbal methods of hypnosis. There
exists some question as to whether or not the drug-induced
state is similar to what we think of as an hypnotic state. We
have touched upon this problem in the chapter on "Methods
of Induction". When a state of being can be defined only in
operational terms and when another state appears to be characterized by similar phenomena, it does not seem to us far-fetched

to conclude the possible existence of at least a large area of overlapping between them. Actually, a description of the "working through" of a traumatic war experience under the influence of one of the barbiturates is indistinguishable from a description of the abreactive process in hypnosis. The same peculiar revivification of the experience with hypermnesia, hallucinatory experiences, and a complete return of the attendant emotion is seen in both. Thus Grinker and Spiegel (158) describe the release of repressed emotion under the influence of sodium pentothal (with the aid usually of verbal stimulation) as the same kind of dramatic return to the traumatic episode described by Hadfield, Brown and others. The experience with abreaction in what has been called "narco-analysis" (180) is similar.

We include the abreactive aspect of Grinker and Spiegel's "narcosynthesis" in this section because we feel that that portion of the psychotherapy is closely allied to the cathartic release in hypnosis. It should be added, however, that the total therapy of "narcosynthesis" goes far beyond a simple abreaction of the experience. The therapist often attempts to allay the patient's anxiety even during the violent re-living, sometimes giving consolation, and again reassuring support. When this is taken together with the fact that psychotherapeutic interviews are then held in the normal state in order to integrate this material with the waking ego, we see that the total therapy is actually closer, in principle, to the methods of hypno-analysis than to the technique of abreaction. It is a dynamic psychotherapy broadly oriented by psychoanalytic theories and techniques.

Some of the advantages and disadvantages of drug adjuvants have been mentioned in Chapter Two. We feel that the most important objection to stimulating chemically the abreaction of the traumatic experience lies in the fact that one runs the risk of setting off a process that is, in a sense, set apart from the current ego orientation of the patient. Although Grinker and Spiegel have devised excellent techniques for circum-

venting this difficulty, the fact remains that a radical physiological alteration of consciousness takes place, more radical
than that in hypnosis, and less controllable (except again, by
other chemical means, e.g., the use of benzedrine to keep
the patient awake).

Hadfield (162) has discussed this problem on the basis of
his experience with the treatment of the psychiatric casualties
of World War II. He believes that the barbiturates may be
used as an aid in psychotherapy but that they should not be
substituted for the "more delicate psychological methods" of
free association and "hypno-analysis". He points out that when
the drug succeeds in stimulating the abreactive process, this
experience is often forgotten by the patient and must be again
"worked through" in the normal state. Thus, the synthesizing
aspect of the psychotherapy is often, of necessity, temporally
and psychologically divorced from the re-living of the repressed affect.

Hadfield emphasizes that it is not a matter of determining
to use one technique or the other, but that each has its specific
applicability and that the therapist who is confronted with war
casualties should have both at his command.

We conclude this section with an evaluation of the abreactive
technique. Its primary advantage over both types of direct
suggestion is that it is an "uncovering" rather than a suppressive method. Moreover, it has been our experience and that
of others (130) (159) that the relief of acute symptoms may
follow directly upon the re-living of the pertinent traumatic
episodes. This has seemed particularly true for the war neuroses,
although it is by no means restricted to them. Thus, it is a
relatively brief method. It is, in addition, a technique which
may yield good clinical results even when applied by therapists who have not had intensive training in the methods of
modern psychotherapy. This does not imply that the abreactive
method may be employed by persons who have no orientation
in the problems of psychodynamics; for if the material brought
by the patient is regarded simply as a mechanical release of

emotion and is not integrated with his total personality, the re-living experience may be harmful to the patient. However, the kind of sympathetic reassurance which seems of paramount importance here is a psychotherapeutic technique that requires less specialized training than the technique of directly suggesting a change in underlying attitudes or of hypno-analysis. These methods require a more specific and deeper understanding of the total personality of the individual.

The limitations of the abreactive method lie first in the fact that, in general, a deep hypnosis is required before the typical "re-living" can occur. This has been less true for the war neuroses in which it appears that the repressed emotion is closer to the surface. Secondly, this method is largely a "symptom-treatment" if it is restricted to abreaction alone. The therapy starts with the symptom and tries to trace it back, allowing for few detours. The variety of insight which the patient achieves by such an approach is thus relatively shallow and one cannot feel that the cure is rooted in personality changes sufficiently deep to provide a reliable equilibrium. Here again, one must emphasize that this is an argument based more on theoretical considerations than on established empirical findings, for many abreactive "cures" are permanent.

5. *The Use of Specialized Hypnotic Techniques.*

Although all methods of hypnotherapy involve the use of one or another of hypnotic techniques and phenomena, we are considering this approach as distinct from the other methods because it has been used beyond the point where hypnosis is merely a catalyst or an adjuvant. The variegated phenomena of hypnosis are used here as the nucleus of the therapeutic leverage in a way which demarcates this method from the others. Highly differentiated techniques are employed and the fact of the patient's being in hypnosis is therapeutically exploited to its limits; these include not only the standard hypnotic phenomena (hypermnesia, posthypnotic suggestion, and so forth) but also more specialized procedures.

For example, it has been established that a patient in hypnosis will automatically write out, if properly instructed, information that is inaccessible to direct awareness. Muhl (198) has used such "automatic writing" to recover childhood memories. A similar approach is the attempt to recover normally inaccessible material by asking a patient in hypnosis to fix his gaze on some neutral, ambiguous field, such as a light-bulb, a glass ball, or a mirror, and to tell him he will experience vivid visual images related to the problems under investigation. This is a kind of "projective technique" in which the patient's projection takes on a hallucinatory vividness. It is usually referred to by the ancient expression "crystal gazing", a phenomenon known to occur spontaneously among "mediums". Both Muhl and Prince (207) investigated this device.

Another important specialized technique of hypnosis is the artificial "regression" of the patient to an earlier time in his life. Phenomenally, the patient "returns" in his behavior and in his reported subjective experience to the suggested age-level. Erickson, in his experimental work on hypnotically induced blindness (142) and deafness (144) has described the procedures whereby the subject is first disoriented with regard to current time-place relationships before new orientations are suggested. In a clinical report (147) he points out the necessity for inducing successive amnesias for the current date, week, month, and year before suggesting that the patient subjectively return to an earlier time. Although there has been much heated controversy regarding the precise nature of such a regression (206) (249) (160), it has been included as one of the tools of hypnotherapy.

Other specialized hypnotic techniques include: the direct suggestion of dreams either in the hypnotic state or posthypnotically as part of the patient's natural sleep; the artificial implantation of a temporary conflict;[25] the use of various de-

---

[25] Eisenbud (140) has used this technique in an experimental case study on the "psychology of headache".

vices to obtain material inaccessible to direct awareness (telling the patient he will see written on a blackboard a single word which will provide a clue to the problem at hand, suggesting vivid visual images, and the like).

Although Janet, Prince, Sidis, Muhl, Wells, and others have explored some of these specialized techniques, the most extensive therapeutic applications of them have been made by Erickson. Combining a unique inventiveness with a shrewd and intuitive grasp of the patient's psychological status, he uses these methods as the essential levers of his therapy.

In a paper written with Kubie (147) Erickson reports the cure of an "acute hysterical depression" in three hypnotic sessions. The patient had become so gravely ill that, after her failure to respond to psychoanalytic treatment,[26] several consultants had favored her commitment to a state hospital. As a last resort, hypnotherapy was tried. From a fragmentary history obtained from the patient's roommate, Erickson concluded that the depression was the result of deep feelings of guilt and terror connected with a sexual experience which had directly preceded the acute symptoms.

In order temporarily to allay her fears, he gave her permission in a deep hypnosis "to forget absolutely and completely many things". The authors point out that this was a radical departure from the technique of psychoanalysis inasmuch as repression was explicitly encouraged by the therapist. Next, she was "regressed" to a period of early adolescence during which her mother had died. Erickson identified himself at first with the prim, moralistic standards of the girl's mother and having established this identity was able to extend "what the mother might have said had she lived"; this extension included permission and encouragement to lead a normal adult sexual life. The patient responded well and shortly was en-

[26] Hypnosis has sometimes been used to render a patient accessible where other techniques have failed. After contact with the patient has been established this may be followed by a course of psychotherapy conducted either in the normal or in the hypnotic state. Brenman and Knight have reported two cases of this kind (123) (124).

tirely symptom-free. Although this account does not do justice to the nuances of procedure, it illustrates the unorthodox and skillful use made by Erickson of hypnosis.

In his report on "The Investigation of a Specific Amnesia" (143) he employs almost every possible technical device, including free association, automatic writing, crystal gazing, dream suggestion, underlining significant letters, and so forth. He succeeded finally in recovering the amnesia by asking the patient to do automatic writing under special circumstances. In a case of a young woman afflicted with an "obsessional phobia" (146), the symptoms disappeared after a few hours of communication with an "unsuspected dual personality" by means of automatic writing and the production of visual images by use of a mirror. Erickson and Kubie (148) report also the use of automatic drawing as an aid in the relief of a state of acute "obsessional depression". This is a representative sampling of the case reports.

Although, from the point of view of varieties of hypnotherapy, it suffices to characterize this approach as that which makes the most consistent use of specialized hypnotic techniques, it is of perhaps greater importance to note the way in which these techniques are applied. It is as if they are used as the "heavy artillery" of a specific strategy, planned to outwit the unconscious of each patient. Before the therapist attempts to manipulate the conscious or unconscious forces in the patient, he conceives a general picture of their current distribution and then applies pressure at those points that seem to him crucial. Thus, in the case of hysterical depression, the therapeutic effort was at first oriented around the aim of reinforcing repression rather than resolving it; and only then was a strong attempt made to manipulate the girl's attitudes.

The advantage of this approach lies in the fact that it makes possible, at least in certain kinds of acute, circumscribed problems, a dramatic and rapid cure. However, because its efficacy is largely dependent on the subtle strategies involved, it is as yet an unsystematized method dependent almost entirely on the personal intuition of the therapist. It is thus exceedingly difficult to communicate as a hypnotherapeutic approach and remains a more or less unique phenomenon, unrelated to a formulated psychopathology and, accordingly, closer to art than to science. Whereas all of the foregoing is true, to a degree, of all methods of psychotherapy, it seems to be the essential characteristic of this approach.

Erickson and Kubie have formulated in their discussions (146) (147) the essential problems regarding the "mechanism of cure" in connection with this type of psychotherapy. They say: "It faces us with the question: if recovery can take place with the gain of such rudimentary insight, what then is the relationship between unconscious insight, conscious insight, and the process of recovery from a neurosis?" This is a vexed question in any form of psychotherapy. One might well ask for the "mechanism of cure" where there exists not even a "rudimentary insight" as in the therapy of direct suggestion of symptom-disappearance, or in the "cures" of Christian Science or of Our Lady of Lourdes. We shall return to this discussion in the concluding chapter.

6. Hypnoanalysis.

Although the hyphenated term "hypno-analysis" was coined by Hadfield (159) to refer to a combination of cathartic hypnosis and "re-education", we shall use the word "hypnoanalysis" to describe those hypnotherapeutic approaches that combine in various ways the techniques of hypnosis with those of psychoanalysis. Actually, there exists a fluid transition between the previously described kinds of hypnotherapy and hypnoanalysis; and it is often difficult to decide to which of the six categories a given approach belongs.

For example, Erickson (145) (146) (147) (148) who frequently collaborates with psychoanalysts in his hypnotherapeutic work, often utilizes the insights of psychoanalysis. Yet the essential nature of the treatment and its duration is usually significantly different from the typical course of a hypnoanalysis. He customarily places but little emphasis on the standard psychoanalytic techniques; and reports the disappearance of symptoms within a comparatively few sessions, whereas hypnoanalytic treatment usually takes from forty to one-hundred hours or more.

The investigations of Lifschitz (183) and Hadfield's later work (159), particularly that with civilian neuroses, fall into a transitional area also. Both trace a symptom back to earlier traumatic experiences in a more systematic and sustained fashion than that usually employed in cathartic hypnosis. Hadfield's psychopathology and his "working concepts" are psychoanalytically oriented, however, whereas Lifschitz, who also calls his technique "hypnoanalysis", is explicitly opposed to psychoanalysis and tries to show that his variety of "hypnoanalysis" disproves many of the basic tenets of psychoanalytic theory.

The term "hypnoanalysis" has been used to refer to somewhat different varieties of hypnotherapy and has been loosely employed to describe a range of therapeutic techniques which includes everything from classical "abreaction" to modified psychoanalytic treatment carried out with the patient in hypnosis.

Although there were a few sporadic attempts as early as 1917 to combine the techniques of psychoanalysis with those of hypnosis (176), the first consistent application of this combined method was in the work of Simmel who explored this approach to some extent in civilian neuroses (225) and on a broader scale in the war neuroses of World War I (226). Simmel had come to the place where his experience dictated a rejection both of "forcible and restrictive methods" and of the technique of symptom-removal by direct suggestion in hypnosis. He says:

> "A medical treatment that is to be effective can only
> be built up on the pathogenesis of a disease. The
> psychopathogenesis of the war neurosis, (and no in-
> telligent man any longer doubts its psychic origin),

obviously can be elucidated only by means of psycho-analysis. It is intelligible that a hospital regime neces-sitating the simultaneous treatment of a large num-ber of cases and calling for rapid curative results, would allow a more extensive individual analysis only in a few cases. On account of this I had from the be-ginning to cut down the length of the treatment. A combination of analytic-cathartic hypnosis with analy-tical conversations during the waking state, and dream interpretation carried out both in the waking state and in deep hypnosis, has given me a method which on an average of two or three sittings brought about re-lief of the symptoms." (226)[27]

During the course of this treatment, the soldier frequently "re-lived" the battle trauma as was described under the sec-tion on cathartic hypnosis. Often this re-enactment with all the attendant emotion and behavior was so violently realistic that it became necessary for Simmel to provide his patients with a dummy, dressed in an army uniform, on which they could safely vent their wrath. He included far more in the treatment, however, than this simple abreactive procedure. The most important psychoanalytic technique which he used in his hypnotherapy was the exploration of the soldier's dreams. He states: "I do not treat any patients whose dreams I do not know."[28] He would ask the patients to continue in hypnosis where their dreams had left off the previous night or to finish during sleep the train of thought begun in hypnosis. He says:

"I recollect a neurotic who suffered from a severe disturbance of speech and also of walking, the result of a spastic paralysis of the legs and muscles of the mouth in consequence of a strong repression of rage. The discharge which took place under hypnosis was so dangerous to those in the vicinity that I had prema-turely to break off the treatment. However, before waking the patient I told him to discharge the un-released part in his dream. I let him sleep alone with

[27] p. 30.
[28] p. 37.

an orderly. In the middle of the night he sprang up
and again lived through an experience of anxiety and
rage accompanied with shouting and raving, and although previously paralyzed he ran down the whole
length of the staircase of the hospital."[29]

Kardiner (174) has also recommended the use of a combined technique for fresh cases of war neurosis and Fisher
(152) has reported favorably on this method as applied to
the casualties of World War II. Although Simmel's pioneer
attempts were stimulated by the immediate practical necessity for a brief yet effective treatment, he recognized the fact
that such a combined method might be of great importance
even in a situation where the emergency was less acute. He
stated: "An analytic cure of the entire personality by a shortened and combined method will have to be reserved for the
psychological clinic of the future."[30]

It was mentioned in the introductory section that during
the early decades of this century, the clinical practice of hypnosis was largely abandoned by psychoanalysts. This meant that
psychiatrists working with hypnosis either were unconcerned
with the psychoanalytic approach or were opposed to psychoanalytic theory. Thus, there was no avenue whereby a "combined method" might be systematically evolved. Schilder's
work was a notable deviation from this general trend (218).
Recently, there have been renewed attempts to study the potentialities of "hypnoanalysis" as a shortened form of psychotherapy and to investigate the hypnotic relationship from a
psychoanalytic point of view. Speyer and Stokvis (230) refer
to Carp's suggestion of the possibility of shortening psychoanalytic treatment by the introduction of hypnotic techniques.
Fervers (151) has taken the same position, placing special emphasis on the character of hypnotic dreams. He reports that
these are usually less disguised than normal dreams. This is
in line with Kubie's work on the hypnagogic reverie (275).

[29] p. 38.
[30] p. 31.

Lindner (184), who has recently reported on the hypnoanalysis of a "criminal psychopath", uses the psychoanalytic technique of free association until he encounters serious resistance. Then he puts the patient into a deep hypnosis in order to obtain the material which the patient has been withholding.

While the patient is in a state of deep hypnosis, he may be regressed or instructed to have hypermnesic recall of the repressed material with the suggestion of posthypnotic amnesia. Lindner's patient was thus able to recover a memory of parental intercourse which he had observed presumably during his first year of life, a memory that was crucial in the elucidation of the meaning of a visual disturbance in this patient. In this case and, according to Lindner, in other patients treated by this variety of hypnoanalysis, the recovery of such a repressed memory in deep hypnosis is shortly followed by spontaneous recall of the same memory in the normal state "if it is memorially valid and not a screen-memory."[31] He says:

> "Apparently the mechanism involved is that of a subliminal appreciation by the organism of diminished 'need' for preserving secrets. In spite of the complete induced amnesia[32]—which can be proved beyond question—the material which resisted disclosure actually flows as smoothly posthypnotically as if no reluctance against its production had ever been present. This single benefit of hypnoanalysis is perhaps responsible for the saving of more than half of the total treatment-time. It effectively counters the already-noted objection that the total personality rarely if ever participates in the disclosures made under hypnosis, and removes what was perhaps the only objection to the employment of hypnosis in the treatment of psychogenic disorders that ever counted for very much in an academic or practical sense."

[31] p. 21.

[32] Lindner suggests amnesia for the memory recovered in hypnosis and finds that despite the success of this suggestion, the same memory very soon appears in free association in the waking state.

The technique of introducing a hypnoidal or hypnotic state in order to penetrate to hitherto inaccessible material has also been employed by Kubie (180). The specific method of induction, devised in collaboration with Margolin, was fully described in Chapter Two (63). We mention it here because its therapeutic application is closely allied to the techniques of hypnoanalysis under discussion.

It is of historical interest to note that the approach, involving the use of hypnosis when gaps in the material are noted, was used by Freud in his early explorations of hypnosis. He said:

> "At first I let the patient relate what was known to her, paying careful attention wherever a connection remained enigmatical, or where a link in the chain of causation seemed to be lacking. Later, I penetrated into the deeper strata of memory by using for those locations hypnotic investigations or a similar technique." (125)[33]

An investigation of hypnoanalysis, its specific applicability, and its limitations, is currently in progress at the Menninger Clinic. In a preliminary report on this work, Gill and Brenman (156) have described their technique in a case of anxiety hysteria as consisting largely of "directed association" conducted with the patient in deep hypnosis. When in the course of the psychotherapy a question was reached which the patient was unable to answer or to which her answer was unenlightening to the therapist, the general formula applied was: "I will count to a certain number and when I reach that number you will tell me the first thing that occurs to you in connection with so-and-so." They also describe other variants of directed association. In addition they utilized various forms of the specialized hypnotic techniques described under Section 5. They describe a portion of this procedure as follows:

> "On a number of occasions, the patient was told that she would have a dream in connection with a

[33] p. 99.

certain problem and this suggestion was almost always successful. On several occasions the patient was made in hypnosis to complete an incomplete dream action. In one dream, for example, she searched through an entire house, though she didn't know what she was looking for. The last place in which she was going to look was the basement. But as she began to go down the stairs she awoke in terror. In the hypnotic hour she was made to go down into the basement and describe what she found. On one occasion the technique of induced regression to an earlier age was used with rather striking results. The patient was regressed to the age of five. We asked her where babies came from. She told us that babies were vomited up but refused to tell her theory as to how they were made. That night she had a dream which was a repetition of an experience at the age of five, in which she had been told of fellatio by a little girl friend. She then told us that it was this memory that she had refused to communicate while she was regressed."

The authors felt that that aspect of the patient's production that involved her strong positive or negative feelings toward the therapist (usually a re-statement of attitudes previously experienced toward parents or surrogate figures, and referred to by psychoanalysts as "transference material") was an important part of the hypnoanalytic treatment. They distinguish between the transference phenomena that are concomitant with the patient's being in the hypnotic state from those that were dealt with in the psychotherapy.

Another case in this preliminary series was reported by Brenman and Knight (123). They describe a case of "hysterical psychosis" in a seventy-one-year-old woman treated by free association in hypnosis combined with several specialized hypnotic techniques (inducing vivid visual images, the revivification of earlier emotional experiences, and so forth). The essential difference between the approach used here and that used in the case described above lay in the fact that no significant "transference phenomena", in the psychoanalytic sense, were manifestly utilized in the treatment.

The variety of modifications of technique described demonstrates that in hypnoanalysis there may be a great number of permutations of the combination of hypnosis with psychoanalysis, with the accent on one or more of the psychoanalytic techniques in one case and on hypnotic devices in another; the common element lies in the fact that hypnosis is used in all instances to circumvent resistances and that psychoanalytic theory and practice provide a constant frame of reference.

Of all the methods of hypnotherapy, hypnoanalysis is the youngest and thus the least widely employed. It is our opinion, however, that it holds the greatest promise for a shortened method of psychotherapy which, nevertheless, retains the crucially important factor of "insight" as a mechanism of cure. It is too early to say in which cases this method will find its greatest value. Thus far, it would appear that it may be used successfully with a wide variety of emotional illnesses. Lindner (184) has studied its use in psychopathic personalities, hysterical somnambulism, frigidity, bronchial asthma, alcoholism, kleptomania, homosexuality, and anxiety neurosis. In general, he reports good therapeutic results.

Investigators at the Menninger Clinic, working in close cooperation with psychoanalysts, have had therapeutic success with hypnoanalysis in cases of anxiety hysteria, hysterical somnambulism, hysterical psychosis, several neurotic depressions, psychogenic reactions to pregnancy, and conversion hysteria. In one case of conversion hysteria the hysterical symptoms promptly disappeared, but the subsequently discovered character disorder required as long a period of treatment as such a problem usually requires in psychoanalysis.

No conclusions can be drawn from these cited cases because they are too few. The fact that a variety of mental illnesses has been successfully treated by hypnoanalysis suggests that its applicability may be wide. Further research will delineate the specific areas of greatest usefulness of this kind of hypnotherapy.[34]

[34] Farber and Fisher (150) have recently reported experiments that show the greater accessibility of unconscious material when the patient is in hypnosis.

The first obvious advantage of hypnoanalysis is that it is, in contrast to direct suggestion, an "uncovering" rather than a "covering-up" psychotherapeutic technique.[35] It shares this advantage with the cathartic method but goes beyond the latter in that it does not rely on an automatic readjustment of psychic forces by dint of the re-living of a traumatic experience, but involves a conscious attempt to integrate the abreacted experience into the total personality through "insight". We have seen that almost all the investigators using hypnoanalysis today are oriented in psychoanalytic psychiatry. It is possible, of course, for followers of other schools of psychological analysis and psychodynamics to combine their particular psychotherapeutic approaches with the techniques of hypnosis. But the orientation of hypnoanalysis within a systematized psychopathology is necessary to provide a "direction" which goes beyond an intuitive but essentially blind production of therapeutic results.

Although it is a relatively brief method of psychotherapy in contrast to psychoanalysis, it is far more time-consuming than any of the hypnotherapeutic approaches previously discussed. The therapist is more passive than in the other methods of hypnotherapy and permits the patient far greater latitude in choosing the "topics" for discussion. He does not create a role for himself but allows the patient to fantasy one or more roles for him, as in psychoanalysis. This may be considered a disadvantage viewed against the other therapeutic applications of hypnosis. The justification for the additional time-expenditure lies in the assumption that a more thorough exploration will result in a more complete and lasting cure.

A more significant disadvantage of this technique lies in the fact that it requires far more training in the psychology of

---

[35] Since the first publication of this monograph there has appeared an important and valuable book in the field: *Hypnoanalysis*, by Lewis R. Wolberg. New York: Grune and Stratton, 1945. This book presents the hypnoanalysis of a schizophrenic in which psychoanalytic and many specialized hypnotic techniques are used. It also discusses problems of transference, resistance, interpretation, and so forth, in hypnoanalysis.

personality and in the general techniques of psychotherapy than does any of the other methods of hypnotherapy. The hypnoanalyst must be familiar with the problems of psychodynamics if he is to have any means of adequately handling the material brought by the patient in a hypnoanalytic treatment.

Whereas an internist with little or no training in psychiatric problems could successfully use the methods of prolonged hypnosis, direct suggestion of symptom-relief, or of abreaction, he could not use either the method directed against underlying attitudes or that of hypnoanalysis, because both hinge on a deeper understanding of the psychological problems of the patient.

We have seen in this presentation of the therapeutic applications of hypnosis that there are at least six different methods of hypnotherapy, that some of them simply utilize the hypnotic relationship in an attempt to suppress symptoms and that others use it to explore the etiology of the illness in an effort to bring about insight in the patient.

7. Supposed Dangers of Hypnotherapy.

It is curious that although almost every discussion of hypnotherapy in the literature includes a section on the "dangers of hypnosis", there is universal agreement that, in the words of Neustatter (205), "the dangers of hypnotism, like the reports of Mark Twain's death, are greatly exaggerated". With a very few exceptions to be mentioned, writers on the subject point out that there is no evidence for a belief that hypnotherapy may have deleterious effects on the patient.

Schultz (220), who made the most systematic investigation of reports of "injuries due to hypnosis", found that most of these had occurred where hypnosis had been used for entertainment or to satisfy the curiosity of an amateur. Even these injuries were shown to be amenable to appropriate treatment. Moll (194) says that he has never seen anyone become disturbed as a result of being hypnotized unless "exciting suggestions" were given irresponsibly, without taking care to restore the person to the normal state gradually. He adds that the possible danger of bringing about a too easy susceptibility to hypnosis may be prevented by telling the patient in hypnosis that no one will be able to hypnotize him against his will, that he will never experience "hypnotic phenomena" in the normal state, and so forth. Bernheim (119) gives substantially the same discussion.

Janet (172) has gone so far as to say that he even regards it as "unfortunate" that there is so little danger attached to the use of hypnosis. He says:

> "I say 'unfortunate' for the reason that a medicament is not really potent unless it is able to be dangerous on occasions; and it is very difficult to think of any method of treatment which would be efficacious although it could never by any possibility do harm. The dangers attaching to the use of a poisonous drug make it necessary that we should study with great care how to administer it, and in what doses; but the fact that the drug is poisonous is the primary indication that it is powerful. We can hardly say as much of suggestion and of experimental hypnosis, for, even in bad hands, suggestion and hypnotism do not seem to have been able to do much harm."[36]

There is general agreement that care should be taken to separate clearly the hypnotic and the normal states so that the patient does not carry over into his daily life the reactions that occur in hypnosis.

In the more recent literature two major dangers have been discussed: 1) the possibility that the patient may develop an undue subordination to the therapist (134) (178) (219); 2) the danger of exacerbating an incipient psychosis (164) (182). With regard to the first, Schilder and Kauders (219) say that although this danger does exist, it is not certain that this is a more prominent pitfall in hypnotherapy than in other forms of psychotherapy, especially psychoanalysis. The second

[36] p. 236.

seems to be of greater significance. Heyer (164) feels strongly that hypnotherapy is contraindicated in cases where the hypnotic experience may be "pathologically elaborated"; and Levine (182) points out that it may be used to crystallize a developing delusion in an incipient schizophrenia and should therefore not be employed in such cases. Heyer remarks further that it should not be employed in the "circular insanities" inasmuch as a failure will tend to accentuate the trend toward depression.

Schilder and Kauders warn against the mixture of experimental with therapeutic hypnosis. They feel that the patient immediately recognizes the experimental character of such attempts and that this prejudices the therapeutic end.

It would appear that in general the actual dangers of employing hypnosis are slight when the fundamentals of responsible inter-personal relationships are observed by the hypnotherapist; but that there is a contraindication when the patient is on the verge of a psychosis.

The objection has been made that hypnotherapy always runs the risk of "by-passing" the resistances and defenses of the patient, with the result that the ego of the patient is not sufficiently involved in the treatment to effect a genuine reintegration of the personality, and that one obtains unstable symptom-relief. Although this objection holds true to a large extent in the methods of "direct suggestion", we have seen that in the method of "abreaction", integration may be achieved by a follow-up of the re-living experience, and that in hypnoanalysis many techniques have been devised to insure the active participation of the total personality (156) (184).

It should be added that in those hypnotherapeutic techniques (like direct suggestion) that produce cures even in the total absence of "insight", the symptom-relief is often maintained where the disorder has been relatively peripheral to the total personality.

CHAPTER FIVE

THE THEORY OF HYPNOSIS

Since this monograph is primarily devoted to a review of the literature on hypnotic therapy, a word of introduction for the advisability of including a section on hypnotic theory may be necessary. Perhaps the most cogent reason is that the manner in which hypnosis has been used—or discarded—by psychotherapists has been significantly influenced by their theoretical conception of the nature of the hypnotic state. Theories of hypnosis differ widely and in general, of course, the particular theory that an investigator holds is one which fits into the general framework of his conception of psychodynamics and psychotherapy. The past few years have seen a re-awakening of interest in developing theories of the hypnotic state, notably by Kubie and Margolin (276) and White (290).

One of the great difficulties here is that it is still highly controversial as to what actually constitutes the hypnotic state, in contrast to the manifestations within it which are the result of suggestion, whether direct or indirect. In other words, what can we find within the hypnotic state which is solely a result of the induction of hypnosis and has not been suggested by the hypnotist?

As early as 1926, Young in reviewing the literature (292) dismissed catalepsy, posthypnotic amnesia, and exclusive rapport of the subject with the operator as integral correlates of the hypnotic state, showing that all these were the results of suggestion and do not necessarily appear if appropriate suggestions are not made. In 1933 Hull (270) did the same with

91

the lowering of sensory threshold, showing that actual measurement fails to reveal a significant change in it from the normal level in the hypnotic state. Ordinarily one attempts to understand a phenomenon by comparing it with similar conditions or states. As will be shown in some detail in what follows, this has also been attempted with the hypnotic state; but there is always the question whether the phenomenon chosen as common to the hypnotic and any other state is actually characteristic of hypnosis or is perhaps only a suggested phenomenon.

For example, the hypnotic phenomenon of catalepsy—the tendency of the subject to maintain an extremity in whatever position it is placed and with less effort than would be required to maintain the position voluntarily—forms an important base of theories attempting to link hypnosis as a physiological state with certain postencephalitic conditions or states. In these theories it is contended that certain of the changes in functioning of the central nervous system produced by the irreversible organic changes due to the encephalitic process are similar to those temporarily produced by the induction of the hypnotic state. But as already stated, Young, Hull, and others find catalepsy to be a suggested and not a spontaneous phenomenon. On the psychological side, the hypnotic state has been linked with hysterical conditions and more specifically with hysterical phenomena like multiple personality, fugue, and conversion symptoms in both the motor and sensory spheres. It is argued that hypnosis is an artificial hysteria and that both are produced by the same psychological mechanisms. But here again the objection is often heard that phenomena like these are, in hypnosis, the result of suggestion. It is agreed by practically all investigators, however, that the response of an individual to a particular suggestion is increased in the hypnotic as compared with the waking state. We reserve this for later discussion.

Theories of hypnosis fall naturally into two major classes, the physiological ones which view hypnosis as an altered condition of the brain, and the psychological ones which see it as a unique interpersonal relationship. Some theories attempt to combine the two points of view, but even in these the two parts of the theory remain quite distinct.

We need spend only a word on the theories that explain hypnosis as resulting from some mysterious emanation from the hypnotist which influences the subject. The earliest form of this theory was the "animal magnetism" of the mesmerists. Even today it has its exponents. Alrutz (251) in Germany claims that a magnetic hypnotic influence perceptible up to a distance of one yard is given off by the human body. One of the more curious manifestations of this idea prevalent around the time of Charcot was the notion of "transference" (unrelated to the modern psychodynamic meaning of transference), according to which the pathological phenomena exhibited by an hysteric could be transmitted to another person by contact, this other person thereby serving as a vehicle of cure. No objective evidence for such emanations has ever been presented.

Early neurophysiological theories of hypnosis as an altered state of the brain were purely speculative and in general based on the idea of some inhibition of central nervous system activity. Heidenhain (267) and Verworn (288) believed hypnosis to be an inhibition of the ganglion cells of the cortex. Dollken (262) conceived of it as a brain anemia with "change in tonus of neural elements". Cappie (258) considered hypnosis a hyperemia of the motor centers with anemia of the rest of the brain.

These neurophysiological theories all imply a similarity between hypnosis and sleep. This presumed relationship continues to be a focal point for theories of hypnosis. Some of the earlier authors contented themselves with calling hypnosis an "artificial sleep", a "sleep-like state", a "state differing from sleep only in that rapport is maintained with the hypnotist", but most tried to give some neurological statement of the condition. Pavlov (280) considered hypnosis a state of inhibition of the brain related to sleep with the inhibition confined to motoric impulses. He spoke of a concentrated excitatory focus

in the central nervous system with surrounding areas of inhibition, and regarded the inhibition as due to a limitation in
either the amount or the type of sensory intake. Biermann
(254) spoke of a waking focus in the cortex of the brain which
continued receptive to stimuli from the hypnotist though the
rest of the brain slept. Isserlin (271) postulated an "island
of wakefulness" in the brain.

Whether or not there is a relationship between hypnosis and
sleep is a much debated point. Those who hold that there is
believe that the hypnotic state is an altered state of consciousness. Most hypnotists believe that the conditions favorable
for the induction of sleep, such as monotonous stimulation, restriction of avenues of stimulation, and so on, are indispensable in the induction of hypnosis. They cite such well-documented phenomena as the possibility of getting into hypnotic
rapport with a sleeper (possible in some cases) without waken-
ing him. But other investigators believe this to be false, and
hold that hypnosis can be induced without any reference to
sleep and without the production of circumstances conducive
to sleep. A particularly strong exponent of this point of view
is Wells (289) who induces "waking hypnosis" and believes that
the lethargic manifestations of hypnosis appear only when they
are suggested by the hypnotist. Even when hypnosis is induced
by suggestions of sleep, the lethargic manifestations can be
entirely abolished in a good subject, so that an observer ig-
norant that the subject is in hypnosis may not suspect anything out of the ordinary.

Attempts to measure physiological processes in hypnosis in
order to determine whether they yield findings similar to
those of the waking or sleeping state have shown conflicting
results, but the bulk of the evidence to date speaks against
hypnosis as a sleep state. Studies of pulse and respiration rates
show no changes from the waking state (273). An experiment
considered by many investigators to be the conclusive one in
the field is that of Bass (252), who demonstrated that the
knee-jerks disappear in sleep but not in hypnosis. He also found

that the motor response to a stimulus in the hypnotic state was the same as that in the waking, and contrasted with that of the sleeping state. One of the reports on the other side is that of Heilig and Hoff (268), who found the response to adrenalin of the hypnotized subject to be the same as that of the sleeper. An objective somatic criterion of hypnosis does not exist. The attempts to use cortical electroactivity as a somatic criterion have yielded contradictory results (277) (278). Stokvis (286) believes that changes in the psychogalvanic reflex come closest to definitively differentiating the hypnotic and waking states.

The modern theory of a sleep center in the neighborhood of the third ventricle has given rise to new forms of the theory of hypnosis as sleep. These are especially advanced by Schilder and Kauders (284) and by Stokvis. The latter believes that the monotonous stimulations of hypnotic induction tire the cortex generally and result in more stimuli going to the sleep center, bringing about an artificial sleep or hypnosis. He gives the same explanation for the fact that people can be hypnotized more easily at night and when they are tired. Stokvis holds that steadily maintained ocular convergence is the best method for inducing hypnosis because of the proximity of the center for convergent gaze to that of the sleep center. He states that in his experience myopes are poorer subjects than others and explains this by pointing to the fact that the resting position of the eyes in myopes is divergent, so that forced convergence is painful and interferes with the attempt to sleep.

Schilder and Kauders believe that certain manifestations of some postencephalitics are due to the same alterations of neurophysiology found in the hypnotic state. They concern themselves particularly with muscular and ocular phenomena and with alterations of consciousness. They believe catalepsy and some types of tremor to be spontaneous manifestations of the hypnotic state in at least some individuals, and regard these motor manifestations as "extrapyramidal release phenomena" analogous to alterations of muscular tone and tremors in some postencephalitics. They relate the altered state of consciousness in hypnosis to the sleep center in the third ventricle and ascribe the lethargy of encephalitics to the same region of the brain. They postulate that vegetative changes are so easily producible in hypnosis because centers for vegetative innervation are present in the same region—third ventricle area and hypothalamus—and this is at least one of the regions whose neurophysiology they hold to be altered in the hypnotic state.

Schilder and Kauders (284) and others find evidence for their view that hypnosis is an altered state of the brain in the hypnotizability of some animals. Whether animal hypnosis is a phenomenon really comparable to human hypnosis is again a moot point. Trömner (287) believes that a decisive differentiating point is that with increasing practice animals become less, humans more, susceptible. Schilder and Kauders (and Stokvis) hold that the essential factor in the production of animal hypnosis is the prevention of the animal from carrying out the righting reflexes which would normally follow from putting the animal into certain positions. They hold that the excitability of righting reflexes is diminished in human hypnosis and that this links it with animal hypnosis. They also report instances in which elicitation of the tonic neck reflexes in human beings (they do not make it clear whether they mean normals or postencephalitics) is accompanied by alterations in the state of consciousness. Stokvis states that he has been able to induce cataplexy in a few of his easily hypnotizable subjects by suddenly frightening them and, regarding cataplexy as due to a lesion in the region of the third ventricle, he finds this another argument for the involvement of this area in hypnosis.

The physiological theories thus far discussed make no attempt to describe the altered physiological state in psychological terms. We shall later see that in theories like those of McDougall, Kubie, and White, physiological factors are stressed, but they are also expressed in psychological terms.

We believe the exposition will be clearer if we turn first to psychological theories of the nature of hypnosis. We find the first milestone to be the concept of suggestion, first systematically elaborated by Braid (255) and later by Bernheim (253). Bernheim went so far as to say that "there is no hypnosis but only suggestion". The great merit of this theory at the time of its proposal was that it proclaimed hypnosis to be a psychological phenomenon in contrast to the theory of Charcot (259) who believed it to be purely somatic. Charcot believed that hypnosis consisted of three well-defined stages which were producible by physical manipulations. Rubbing of the scalp or spine, and loud auditory stimuli were believed to initiate hypnosis while forcibly opening the eyelids of an individual in hypnotic catalepsy was supposed to put him into somnambulism. The views of Bernheim and Charcot were basically opposed in another respect, too. Bernheim believed hypnosis to be producible in normal individuals and a non-pathological phenomenon, whereas Charcot considered that it was pathological and producible only in hysterics. The demonstration by the Nancy School that Charcot was wrong, and that his subjects responded as they did because they believed his manipulations would produce the results they did, was most important in firmly establishing the significance of psychological factors in hypnosis. Charcot's error is one that every investigator of a therapeutic procedure must take into account. He must ask how important a role is played by the patient's belief in the efficacy of the therapy.

The prime difficulty with the concept of suggestion is that it has been elevated to an explanatory role and it is often deemed sufficient to account for a piece of human behavior, whether psychological or physical, by stating that it is the "result of suggestion". While the concept of "suggestion" continues to be used in connection with both hypnosis and other phenomena, its meaning is now considerably altered in that it is considered merely a descriptive term for the fact that an individual responds positively to a particular communication, whether verbal or non-verbal, direct or indirect. All modern investigators recognize that one must go beyond this fact to discover why it is that "suggestions" are accepted.

One must ask whether the hypnotic state facilitates the acceptance of suggestions, which suggestions are especially facilitated, and how it is that the hypnotic state produces these changes in suggestibility. Sidis (285) has attempted to break down the concept of "suggestion" in an effort to give it more specific meaning. He has suggested that a distinction be made between "direct" and "indirect" suggestion: the former refers to direct statements made, for example, to an hypnotic subject; the latter to the introduction of an idea by tricks, disguises, ambiguities, "double-entendres" and the like. Young (293), who has written one of the most searching criticisms of the loose concept of "suggestion", has stated:

"Suggestion is definitely a method of communication of meanings or attitudes, so imparting the 'idea' as to elude rational criticism. *It is a method of indirect appeal to the person to be influenced.* Suggestion has a negative and a positive aspect. The negative aspect consists in inhibiting the action of the more strictly critical intellectual functions in one of two ways: either by so craftily clothing and introducing the communication that its true nature is unrecognized, or by so drugging the critical consciousness—through emotional appeals or through a technique of monotony—that almost any communication will be acceptable. The positive aspect, also, has two sides: the trend may be awakened by the communication, or it may be merely freed by the inhibition of other motives. Although the complete method of suggestion, exemplified best in its professional use in psychotherapy, shows both the inhibiting and the positive aspects, many suggestions manifest mainly one or the other. Some depend on the subtlety of the expression, as in hints and intimations; some depend on the thoroughness of the precursory process of inhibition, as in hypnosis and autosuggestion; still others depend on taking advantage of states of inhibition brought about by chance or by informal means, in order to insinuate the communication, as in crowd appeals, or suggestions given after a good dinner."[37]

The essential point here seems to be the distinctions made between the various kinds of factors which may bring about a condition in which almost any communication will be acceptable. It would appear thus that there may be a significant difference between various methods of "drugging the critical consciousness". For example, the administration of a placebo in the normal state to a patient plays upon his gullibility and presumably would be totally without effect if he recognized its true nature, whereas a direct statement in hypnosis that a symptom will disappear is presumed by Young to be effective because of the "precursory process of inhibition". The further delineation of these distinctions is a task for the future.

Practically all investigators hold hypnosis to be a state of hypersuggestibility, though there are opponents even of this point of view. Brown (257) believes, for example, that in deep hypnosis suggestibility decreases. Hull (270) finds in hypersuggestibility the only specific characteristic of the hypnotic state. He says:

"The only thing which seems to characterize hypnosis as such and which gives any justification to the practice of calling it a 'state' is its generalized hypersuggestibility. The difference between the hypnotic state and the normal one is therefore a quantitative rather than a qualitative one. Responsiveness to suggestions emanating from other people, to 'prestige suggestion', is a very common phenomenon but this is not the distinguishing mark. The essence of hypnosis lies in the fact of change in suggestibility. The experimental fact of a shift in the upward direction which may result from the hypnotic procedure . . . Hypnotic hypersuggestibility has a relative and not an absolute significance."

[37] p. 89.

We may digress here for a moment to consider the controversy between the concepts of autosuggestion and heterosuggestion. Coué and Baudouin revised Bernheim's dictum—"there is no hypnosis; there is only suggestion"—to "there is no suggestion, only autosuggestion". This correction arises in reaction against the earlier concept that the hypnotic subject is a passive automaton blindly responsive to the suggestions of the hypnotist. With the development of our modern understanding of personality as the expression of an individual dynamic interplay of strivings, it has become clear that the hypnotized subject is by no means an automaton, that a suggestion takes effect only if it is consonant with the balance of forces of the individual's strivings, and that his understanding and elaboration of a suggestion are likewise determined by his own personality structure. The attempt to emphasize this truth may be construed as implying that the only kind of suggestion is autosuggestion; but as Schilder and Kauders point out, one could as well say that there is no education but only autoeducation, since it does not matter how much an individual is taught if he does not learn anything.

Although the concept of "suggestion" continues to play an important role even currently, the next significant step in the development of the theory of hypnosis was the concept of dissociation as advanced by Janet (272). The rise and fall of this concept, as well as its extension to include ideas other than those intended by Janet, is well described in an article by White and Shevach (291). Janet was led to his explanation of hypnosis by way of his theory of hysteria, since he regarded hypnosis as an artificially induced hysteria. Janet's idea was that various psychological "systems" could split off from the main psychic stream and exist independently. In some instances, as in hysterical blindness, the dissociated system drops out of function. In others, such as hysterical somnambulism, the dissociated system "takes over" and the rest of the personality ceases to function. This formulation has descriptive value and Janet deserves great credit for being one of the first to really see that ideas and memories can be split off from the stream of consciousness and nevertheless continue to exert influence on behavior; but as an explanatory concept it is vulnerable to two major objections. First of all, the dissociations producible in hypnosis (and in hysteria) do not necessarily follow either natural biological or acquired psychological lines of cleavage, but are subject to the caprice of the hypnotist. While hysterical blindness, for example, can be quite plausibly conceived of as a dissociation of the optic system, it is difficult to see how any natural biological or acquired psychological system can be involved in such hypnotic phenomena as the inability to see one particular person in the room though vision is intact for everything else. Secondly, the concept of dissociation carried with it no explanation of the cause for the dissociation. Janet's concept of dissociation is usually looked upon as a psychological one, but it seems to us that although his clinical descriptions are on the psychological level, his explanation of dissociation was a purely speculative neurophysiological energy theory, in which he considered the energy available for psychological synthesis to be deficient and spoke of "psychic hypotension". Despite Janet's acute clinical observation he was led to a barren speculation in terms of nervous energy, instead of to a psychopathological theory of conflict such as was evolved by Breuer and Freud (256) from similar case material.

Closely allied to the concept of dissociation are the intellectualistic theories of suggestion and hypnosis. By "intellectualistic" we mean theories that fail to take into account motivational factors. One of the best examples is McDougall's (279). He regards hypnosis as a state of hypersuggestibility and defines suggestion as the acceptance of an idea without adequate logical grounds. He believes that it is accepted because it remains isolated, that it is dissociated, and is not confronted with other ideas which might modify or contradict it. That this theory, like Janet's, is physiological rather than psychological seems to us evident in the following statement by McDougall:

> "The monotonous stimulations seem to aid in bring-
> ing the whole brain to a quiescent condition by facili-
> tating the continued direction of attention to an
> object or impression of an unexciting, uninteresting
> character, and thereby preventing the free play of
> ideas which otherwise may maintain itself for a con-
> siderable period in the way noted above. In terms of
> neural process we may say the monotonous stimula-
> tion tends to keep some one minor disposition or small
> system of dispositions in dominant activity and keeps
> open this one path of discharge so that this one chan-
> nel constantly draining off on the sensory side of the
> brain the supply of neurokyme, depresses or tends to
> prevent the activity of all others . . . We must re-
> member that in the waking state of the brain all dispo-
> sitions and systems of disposition are in relation of
> reciprocal inhibitions with one another, so that the
> activity of any one tends to inhibit the activity of any
> other. And we may fairly suppose that between dis-
> positions whose activities underlie incompatible or
> contradictory ideas about any object, this relation of
> reciprocal inhibition is intimate and direct . . . In
> hypnosis, on the other hand, this depressing, weaken-
> ing influence of partial inhibition is abolished or
> diminished in virtue of and in proportion to the de-
> gree of relative dissociation or functional isolation of
> dispositions from one another, since any idea sug-
> gested by the hypnotizer is not only accepted uncriti-
> cally but operates with greater force than any idea
> accepted with conviction in the waking state."[38]

This theory is an advance over the simple suggestion theory in that it stresses psychic interaction and interplay, but it remains on the intellectualistic, ideational level. As we shall see later, however, this is only the first half of McDougall's theory. He was one of the first to formulate a psychological theory of hypnosis which goes beyond the bare statement that "it is only suggestion".

[38] p. 109.

As already indicated in the discussion of autosuggestion, those theories of hypnosis that have been formulated on the basis of our modern conception of personality view the hypnotic state as a set of emotionally imbedded strivings. It is this idea that White (290) states on a descriptive level when he speaks of "hypnosis as a goal-directed striving in which the individual attempts to behave like a hypnotized person as this has been continuously defined by the operator and understood by the subject".

We must ask what are the general and what are the specific aspects of this "definition of the hypnotic state". Is it deeply anchored in an important interpersonal relationship, or is it a relatively superficial behavior pattern learned in the immediate situation?

This really raises the question of why the subject has this wish to behave like a hypnotized person as defined by the hypnotist. An attempt to understand this leads inevitably to a discussion of the nature of the interpersonal relationship between hypnotist and subject. The most searching discussions of this topic have been psychoanalytically oriented. Psychoanalytic theories of hypnosis are built on the premise that instinctual wishes of the subject are elicited and given some gratification by the hypnotic situation. They view hypnosis as a variety of transference, meaning that the subject acts under the dominance of unconscious, infantile, instinctual drives. Ferenczi (264) viewed the hypnotic relationship as a reactivation of the Oedipus complex with the subject standing in a child-to-parent relationship toward the hypnotist. He differentiated "maternal" and "paternal" forms of hypnosis, the first based on love and the second on fear.

The next important psychoanalytic contribution to the theory of hypnosis was presented by Freud in *Group Psychology and the Analysis of the Ego* (265). Freud compares hypnosis to being in love. He says: "There is the same humble subjection, the same compliance, the same absence of criti-

cism toward the hypnotist just as toward the loved object."[39]
The hypnotist steps into the place of the "ego-ideal" and the
testing of reality becomes altered in accordance with the
suggestions of the hypnotist. "The hypnotic relation is the devotion of someone in love to an unlimited degree but with
sexual satisfaction excluded." In addition to this comparison
with being in love, however, Freud stresses the "element of
paralysis derived from the relation between someone with
superior power and someone who is without power and help-
less."[40] The explanation of this last is derived from Freud's
conception of hypnosis as "a group of two". Referring to the
"uncanny" aspects of hypnosis, he suggests that the uncanny
is something "old and familiar that has undergone repression".[41] He proceeds to trace the "uncanny" and coercive characteristics of the phenomena of group psychology and hypnosis
to their origin from the primal horde, conceiving of the relation
between subject and hypnotist as well as that between group
and leader as a reactivation of that of the individual member
of the primal horde to the primal father. It is this primal relationship which is the "something old and familiar that has
undergone repression". Without attempting to discuss this
latter part of the theory any further, we see that Freud views
hypnosis as a transference relationship involving libidinal and
submissive instinctual strivings, in a sense a combination of
Ferenczi's "mother" and "father" hypnosis. As a logical corol-
lary of Freud's theory of hypnosis follows his definition of
suggestion: "A conviction which is not based upon perception
and reasoning but upon an erotic tie."[42] He states that he dis-
agrees here with Bernheim who considered suggestion as not
capable of further explanation. As is well known, the term
"erotic" is used in a broad sense in psychoanalytic theory, and
thus can cover both the libidinal and submissive aspects of
hypnosis. While the psychoanalytic theory of hypnosis as a

[39] p. 77.
[40] p. 79.
[41] p. 95.
[42] p. 100.

particular transference relationship seems to us an important advance in the understanding of the relationship between hypnotist and subject, its chief failure is that it, like other purely psychological theories, fails to account for the specificity of the hypnotic state.

These libidinal and submissive strivings appear—as Freud himself says in comparing the hypnotic state to love and the behavior of people in groups—in other conditions too. We are not told how hypnosis is specifically characterized.

McDougall denies the existence of libidinal drives in hypnosis, but considers the hypnotic state an interpersonal relationship based on the "instinct of submission". It is this explanation of hypnotic "rapport" which the second half of his theory develops. Rivers (282), likewise rejecting the libidinal forces, but impressed by the relationship between hypnotic and group phenomena, derives hypnosis from the "herd instinct".

Schilder has made important contributions to the psychoanalytic theory of hypnosis. He bases his considerations on bodily responses of the subject such as the "glance of surrender", trembling, and hysteriform rigidities, typical verbalizations of subjects in hypnosis such as a "delightful sense of fatigue", typical fears and fantasies about hypnosis held by normal people, the typical equation by schizophrenics of hypnosis and being influenced sexually, and material obtained in psychoanalysis of people who had previously been hypnotized.

Schilder emphasizes the varieties of libidinal relationship that may exist between subject and hypnotizer. Homosexual as well as heterosexual strivings appear. He says:

> "We must be mindful of the fact that the sexual constitution of the individual finds an expression in the nature and form of the hypnosis. Persons strongly disposed to love, persons with the tendency to fixate love objects powerfully, customarily are easily inducted into profound hypnosis. Hysterical individuals with a strong tendency for object fixation as a rule are particularly susceptible to hypnosis, while the hyp-

nosis in the case of compulsion neurotics frequently encounters difficulties which is connected with the sadistic attitude of the compulsive neurotics toward their love objects."[43]

In addition to the factors already delineated, Schilder emphasizes the identification the patient makes with the hypnotist. The patient is able to realize his infantile fantasies of power, magic, and the omnipotence of thought and words, by identifying himself with the hypnotist to whom he grants these powers. Schilder also discusses the psychology of the hypnotist, and finds that the hypnotist must have an unconscious wish for magical power and sexual domination of the patient.

> "It is worthy of note that an unsuccessful attempt at hypnosis produces in the hypnotizer a feeling of personal disappointment, which far transcends those bounds that would express a mere natural interest in the business at hand. To be sure all these experiences will, in the case of the hypnotizer, lie far out in the periphery of his experience."

Jones (274) stresses narcissism in his discussion of "suggestion". He finds:

> "Suggestion (is) essentially a libidinal process; through the unification of the various forms and derivatives of narcissism the criticizing faculty of the ego-ideal is suspended so that ego-syntonic ideas are able to follow unchecked the pleasure-pain principle in accordance with a primitive belief in the omnipotence of thought."

Rado (281) discusses in a rather technical way the metapsychology of hypnosis and particularly the mechanism of cure in suggestive and cathartic hypnosis. He believes that in hypnosis as used in these ways a transference neurosis is set up, just as it is in psychoanalytic treatment, but that here the transference remains unresolved, so that the patient periodically re-lives the transference fantasy which is responsible for his cure.

[43] p. 38.

One of the most recent theories of hypnosis, and one which attempts to combine physiological and psychological factors, has been formulated by Kubie and Margolin (276). In this theory, transference factors are given somewhat less importance than in the usual psychoanalytic theory, and physiological factors are stressed. They make a sharp division between the induction of hypnosis and the established hypnotic state. They consider the induction phase of hypnosis a condition of partial sleep in which the nuclear phenomenon is the restriction of sensory-motor relationships between subject and outside world. Postulating that our differentiation of self and outside world is chiefly dependent upon multiple avenues of sensory intake, they further describe this stage as a blurring of the boundaries between the ego and the outside world as well as between "ego past" and "ego present". They regard immobility and monotony as the chief factors in bringing about the induction of hypnosis. They agree that during the induction of hypnosis a "constellation of conscious and unconscious attitudes arises between the hypnotist and the subject in which manifold libidinal displacements and substituted object relationships (i.e., transference phenomena) are active", but they state that "the maneuvers of the hypnotist are designed to concentrate the subject's attention on one field of *sensation* and to withdraw attention from all others". During the induction they believe there takes place a psychic incorporation of the hypnotist into the subject. In the established hypnotic state there is "an extensive carry over (of the transference relationship) from the prehypnotic (presumably induction phase) relationship into the content of the hypnotic state, comparable precisely to the carry-over into the content of any dream of the residues from the emotionally incomplete experiences of the preceding day . . . in the fully developed stage, a diffusion (expansion) of sensorimotor relations occurs with a retention of the dominant but repressed link to the incorporated figure of the hypnotist". For Kubie and Margolin, despite the transference phenomena, hypnosis is only a special variety of an extension of the normal psychophysiological process of maximal attention, which "should be attainable by simple physiological procedures, without the agency of suggestion or even of any human contacts". They state that in a subsequent communication they will offer experimental evidence for this contention.

Freud (265) likewise views the hypnotic process as one of maximal attention, but in his theory, the attention must be directed to the *hypnotist,* not as in Kubie's and Margolin's theory to "one field of *sensation"*. Freud says:

> "Hypnosis can . . . be evoked . . . by fixing the eyes upon a bright object or by listening to a monotonous sound. This is misleading and has given occasion to inadequate physiological theories. As a matter of fact, these procedures merely serve to divert conscious attention and to hold it riveted. The situation is the same as if the hypnotist had said to the subject: 'Now concern yourself exclusively with my person; the rest of the world is quite uninteresting.' It would of course be technically inexpedient for a hypnotist to make such a speech; it would tear the subject away from his unconscious attitude and stimulate him to conscious opposition. The hypnotist avoids directing the subject's conscious thoughts towards his own intentions, and makes the person upon whom he is experimenting sink into an activity in which the world is bound to seem uninteresting to him; but at the same time the subject is in reality unconsciously concentrating his whole attention upon the hypnotist, and is getting into an attitude of rapport, of transference on to him. Thus the indirect methods of hypnotizing, like many of the technical procedures used in making jokes, have the effect of checking certain distributions of mental energy which would interfere with the course of events in the unconscious, and they lead eventually to the same result as the direct methods of influence by means of staring or stroking."[44]

[44] p. 96.

It is here that Freud believes he has found the key to the relationship between hypnosis and sleep.

> "The command to sleep in hypnosis means nothing more or less than an order to withdraw all interest from the world and to concentrate it upon the person of the hypnotist. And it is so understood by the subject; for in this withdrawal of interest from the outer world lies the psychological characteristic of sleep and the kinship between sleep and the state of hypnosis is based upon it."[45]

As we have seen, it is still an unsettled problem as to whether the relationship between sleep and hypnosis is purely this psychological one postulated by Freud, or whether in hypnosis there are also physiological changes related to the physiological changes occurring in sleep. The evidence from the physiological point of view is contradictory. On the psychological side, phenomena similar to those of sleep can be obtained in hypnotic and hypnoid states. Farber and Fisher (263) have reported on the production of dreams and the ready explanation of their unconscious meaning in hypnosis. The hypermnesia with increased access to repressed material in hypnosis is well-known. Kubie reports that in hypnagogic reverie (275) there is a much-increased intensity, as in dreams, of the sensory components of the images and memories which may flow through the mind. But it seems to us that these phenomena are not decisive in determining whether in hypnosis there is an alteration of the state of consciousness, in the sense in which this is true of sleep. There does seem to be a re-alignment of dynamic relationships within the psyche, but whether this is to be described as an alteration of the state of consciousness is another matter. The precise meaning of "alteration of the state of consciousness" is itself a difficult problem.

Schilder believes that the sleep center in the third ventricle is responsive to psychological as well as physiological stimuli,

[45] p. 98.

that the "sleep wish" is important in both sleep and hypnosis, and that in hypnosis one must distinguish the existence of various egos as the "sleep ego", the "dream ego", and that part of the "waking ego" that is still active.

The apparently well-established enhancement of susceptibility to hypnosis through the use of sedative drugs[46] must also be reckoned with in the formulation of an hypnotic theory. Though not specifically concerned with hypnosis, the recent work of Grinker and Spiegel (266) with intravenous pentothal in treating psychoneurotic combat casualties is important in this connection. Under the influence of pentothal the soldiers re-enacted and abreacted their harrowing experiences in a state apparently very much like that of hypnosis.[47] If it is true that the barbiturates act on the hypothalamic region, this may be another piece of evidence that physiological changes in the region of the hypothalamus and third ventricle do play a role in hypnosis.

In his recently published theory of hypnosis (290), White points out that an adequate theory must account for the fact that the range in which suggestions can be successfully executed is wider in hypnosis than in the waking state, though the field in which hypnosis is successful in contrast to the waking state has been limited and defined. In particular it has been discovered that the more a suggestion deviates from functions under the individual's voluntary control, the less is the degree of success achieved. Memory phenomena, for example, can be manipulated far more easily than the psychogalvanic reflex. In defining a "function under voluntary control", one must carefully distinguish between the direct and indirect methods of fulfilling a suggestion. A subject in hypnosis can make his pulse rate increase, but to do so he has to think of a frightening experience, not of the cardiac muscle. One must also clarify the sense in which a particular suggestion has been successful. For example, if a subject sees everything in a room

[46] See Chapter II.
[47] See Chapter IV.

except one particular person this does not mean that a change takes place somewhere between the retina and the visual cortex, but only that the subject is not *consciously* aware of seeing this particular person. That he is unconsciously cognizant of the person is clear from the way in which he avoids directing his gaze toward or bumping into him.

White suggests that the range of actions accessible to the "hypnotic striving" is increased by way of "some slight degree of functional decortication". He derives this from the "relaxation and the restriction of sensory input . . . conducive to drowsiness . . . (which) may be conceived as a slight lowering of functional level, the effect of which is disinhibitory". He believes that "the operator in hypnosis is indispensable because he prevents the subject's passing from light drowsiness into real sleep and because he maintains a continual motivational pressure, a focal press of dominance".

Again the question arises as to whether this "functional decortication" means an altered state of consciousness. White apparently believes that it does. He himself points out one of the difficulties in the problem by asking whether the soldier who receives a severe wound in battle but feels no pain, and does not even know that he has been wounded until some time later, is in an altered state of consciousness. This temporary anesthesia can be compared to hypnotic anesthesia. Certainly there are vital differences between the soldier's emotional and attentional dispositions in the heat of battle as contrasted with his usual state, but is his state of consciousness altered in either the sense or the direction in which it is altered in the sleep state as contrasted with the waking state?

The last type of theory which we will mention is that of hypnosis as a conditioned reflex. This theory has lately been revived by Salter (283). It was the basis of Hilger's theory (269) in the first decade of this century. In essence it states that since an individual forms associations between words and sensations, the word as a conditioned stimulus can call forth the reaction evoked by the situation that the word describes.

It seems to us that this is a superficial statement of the problem which fails to take into account the specificity of the hypnotic state, the possible physiological basis of hypnosis as a conditioned reflex, or the motivational factors involved in hypnosis.

It may be that conditioned reflexes do play some role in some of the phenomena elicitable in the hypnotic state. Kubie (276) has also suggested that "the subject who has been hypnotized many times inevitably develops certain automatic or conditioned reflexes by which a short-cut is established to the hypnotic state".

To discuss the conditioned reflex theory of hypnosis adequately would raise the whole problem of explaining complex human behavior as conditioned reflexes, a problem which we do not feel it advisable to discuss here.

We have seen that the initial conflict in the theory of hypnosis was between those who ascribed it to the power of the operator and those who viewed it as a change in the subject, with the hypnotist acting only to create the necessary conditions. The next conflict was between those who viewed hypnosis as a somatic change in the subject produced by physical manipulations and those who saw it as a psychological state resulting from the attitude of the subject toward the hypnotist. With the victory of the latter view came the concept of suggestion. The theory of dissociation, while representing an advance in the statement of the psychological problem on a descriptive level, boils down as an explanatory concept to a neurophysiological theory. Both suggestion and dissociation are now reduced to the rank of descriptive rather than explanatory concepts.

The development of modern psychology of the personality has overthrown the idea of the hypnotic subject as an automaton completely subject to the power of the hypnotist, and resulted naturally in the view of the hypnotic state as a goal-directed striving, in which the subject attempts to behave like a hypnotized person as this is "defined by the hypnotist and understood by the subject" (290). The subject's motivations have been variously interpreted by the various theories of conation. It has seemed to us that the most penetrating statements of interpersonal relationship between hypnotist and subject have come from the psychoanalysts. But their theories fail to define the specificity of the hypnotic state. The transference relationships which the analysts describe are present in other interpersonal situations besides hypnosis. It is this that makes necessary the consideration of hypnosis as an altered state of the person. We have presented evidence for and against the possible relationship to sleep of this altered state. Our own impression is that while drowsiness and sleep can be produced by hypnotic suggestion, an alteration of consciousness in the direction of sleep is not a necessary feature of hypnosis. It appears to us that hypnosis may be an altered state only in the sense of an as yet incompletely defined specific constellation of the strivings of the subject, that the transcendence of the normal limits of voluntary control follows from this particular constellation (in a sense analogous to that in which under stress of violent emotion people surpass by a wide margin their usual levels of muscular strength and endurance), and that the elucidation of hypnosis will come from a more complete psychological analysis of this constellation. We should then know how the hypnotist must behave and what the personality of the subject must be in order to bring about the hypnotic state. The psychosomatic phenomena involved in suggestion directed to autonomic functions will of course require more than psychological analysis, but these problems seem to us not specific to hypnosis, but common to all psychosomatic investigation.

CHAPTER SIX

SUMMARY AND STATEMENT OF PROBLEMS

The present review of the literature on hypnotherapy shows that the therapeutic applications of hypnosis, as well as the theories advanced to explain the phenomenon, have reflected, on the whole, the changing concepts of psychology, physiology, and psychopathology. Despite significant advances both in the clinical application of hypnosis and in its theory, most standard psychiatric text-books present hypnotherapy as an approach that is limited to the suppression of symptoms "by command or entreaty".

We have seen that although such suppression of symptoms by direct suggestion is *one* of the methods of hypnotherapy several other techniques are possible. Hypnosis may be used as "prolonged sleep"; it may also serve as a medium whereby direct suggestion can be aimed at underlying attitudes rather than at symptoms; traumatic experiences may be revived and "abreacted" in hypnosis; the specialized techniques of hypnosis may be fully exploited to achieve therapeutic leverage, and finally hypnosis may be combined with psychoanalysis in an effort to bring about "insight" in the patient as well as symptom-relief.

We would like to outline some of the problems that we believe must be tackled if hypnotherapy is to develop its potentialities to the full.

Hypnotizability needs to be studied more extensively and with utilization of the best insights of modern psychiatry. Up-to-date figures on the influence on hypnotizability of age, sex, intelligence, psychiatric status, character type and other fac-

114

tors are urgently needed to gain some idea of who is hypnotizable, and of the range in which hypnotherapy may be applicable. Research should be undertaken in the development
of techniques to enhance hypnotizability and to widen the
range of the hypnotizable. Both psychological and physiological factors (like hypnotic drugs) must be considered. The
problem of hypnotizability is intimately connected with that
of the nature of hypnosis. A really adequate knowledge of
who is hypnotizable should offer clues to the nature of the
hypnotic state. A fixed preconceived notion of the nature of
the hypnotic state could be a stumbling block here, inasmuch
as some of the factors which are held in common by those who
are hypnotizable may not be considered in our ordinary psychiatric studies and psychological tests.

Some understanding of the nature of the hypnotic state may
be gained from prolonged study of cure by hypnoanalysis
where the aim is not only therapeutic but also an attempt to
analyze the hypnotic state.

Studies like those proposed by Kubie (294)—in which psychophysiological states, resembling hypnosis but without the
transference phenomena of hypnosis, are produced—should
add much to our understanding of the nature of hypnosis. It
is probably premature to say so without having seen the data,
but we feel that the danger exists in such studies of the experimenter overlooking *himself* as hypnotist even though he
ostensibly does nothing but hook up the apparatus. The problem is similar to that of presumed autohypnosis in primitives,
where the hynotist may really be the fantasied tribal god or
some analogous figure.

Out of a suggestion by Schilder (295) comes a problem
which seems to us worthy of serious consideration. Schilder
believes that there is no necessary relationship between the
depth of hypnosis, as the concept is ordinarily understood,
and the depth of hypnosis in the sense of the extent to which
the individual's personality is really involved in the hypnotic
state. He says that one individual in the somnambulist stage

may be essentially little involved in the hypnotic state where another individual in a light stage of hypnosis may be deeply involved. Both of these types of depth of hypnosis require much clarification and definition. The traditional stages and depths of hypnosis are static concepts which will require much modification if they are to define the fluid and dynamic state that hypnosis appears to be.

The problem of the depth of hypnosis in the sense of degree to which the personality is involved is closely related to the therapeutic potentialities of hypnosis in a particular individual. We have already seen that there is no necessary correlation between the depth of hypnosis in the traditional sense and its effectiveness as a therapeutic agent in a particular case. Tests for the depth of hypnosis in this new sense may give us far more information about the prognosis with hypnotherapy in a particular case than do the traditional tests. It may be far more useful, for example, to discover if an individual can understand a dream significantly better in the hypnotic than in the waking state, than to see if catalepsy can be successfully suggested.

Many of the problems with which those who are studying "brief psychotherapy" are dealing seem to us to have bearing on hypnotherapy, since hypnotherapy can really be considered one of the techniques of brief psychotherapy. It seems to us that the concept of a hierarchy of psychiatric disturbance in the sense of the degree to which the core of the personality is involved is a useful one. It is difficult to define the concept accurately, but grossly we refer to the difference between a symptom peripheral to the mainstream of the personality and a disturbance of the basic character structure. Perhaps psychiatrists and especially psychoanalysts are not sufficiently flexible in their choice of the variety of psychotherapy for a particular case. In hypnotherapy, for example, hypnoanalysis could be reserved for cases that had either not responded to direct suggestion therapy or that manifestly require more thorough-going treatment.

The psychoneuroses of veterans, a problem looming ever larger on the horizon, seem to offer a special challenge to brief psychotherapy. In many cases, the acute disturbance seems superimposed on a basically adequate adjustment and it would seem reasonable that in such cases techniques of brief psychotherapy, including hypnotherapy, could be successfully employed.

In the traumatic neuroses, in particular, repression as a defense mechanism seems to play an especially important role. All observers agree that the defense which is most characteristically penetrated by hypnosis is repression. Group discussion in the course of research on hypnotherapy at the Menninger Clinic had crystallized the hypothesis that defense mechanisms other than repression may be attacked by hypnosis. We have seen some preliminary evidence that the mechanism of "isolation" may be affected by the hypnotic state. Patients in hypnosis often recall events the details of which they were perfectly familiar with in the waking state but which they now report with much more vivid affect, as though, under the influence of the hypnotic state, content and affect had been reunited.

Both intensive and extensive research is necessary in order to explore the potentialities of hypnosis as a therapeutic agent. Such research, conducted within the framework of a scientific psychopathology, and carried through by a close collaboration between those trained in orthodox techniques of psychotherapy and those exploring untried methods, may result in an important addition to the available tools of clinical psychiatry.

FOUR CASE STUDIES

Treatment of a Case of Anxiety Hysteria by an Hypnotic Technique Employing Psychoanalytic Principles [*]

By Merton M. Gill, M.D.,
and Margaret Brenman, Ph.D.

The patient with whom we worked was a conventional middle-class housewife in her middle thirties who was referred to the Menninger Clinic by an internist who had been unable to find any organic basis for her symptoms. She had been ill periodically for seven years, continuously for two years and with marked exacerbation for the preceding six months. The symptoms which concerned her most were daily nausea and vomiting, severe lower abdominal pain, anxiety and depression and trembling of the left hand. There were numerous other symptoms, including headaches, dysmenorrhea, a fear of falling, palpitation and nightmares in which she saw herself being killed or buried.

She gave her history with the vagueness, the many gaps and the placing of the onset of symptoms by successive stages in the most distant past, which Freud has described as so characteristic of hysteria.

[*] Read before the Joint Session of the American Psychoanalytic Association and the psychoanalytic section of the American Psychiatric Association in Detroit, Michigan, May 12, 1943.
Reprinted from: *The Bulletin of the Menninger Clinic*, 7:163-171, Sept.-Nov., 1943.

Although quite intelligent, the patient had a somewhat child-like naiveté. For example, she engaged other patients in the waiting room in conversation about her symptoms and once queried a stranger just outside the Clinic grounds about the work of the Clinic, saying she wanted to be sure that her money was being well spent. She said she supposed this person was another patient who could give her the benefit of his experience.

The history and psychiatric examination pointed unmistakably to a diagnosis of anxiety hysteria. Psychological test findings supported this diagnosis and though she attained an I.Q. of only 100, it appeared that her effective intelligence was diminished by her great anxiety and preoccupation with fantasy.

Psychoanalysis was impracticable in this case for the same reasons that it is so often impracticable. The patient lived two-hundred miles away; her husband and two children needed her; she was in poor circumstances. She was very eager for help, however, and it was decided to determine whether she would be suitable as a case in the hypnosis research project.

The patient's degree of hypnotizability was determined first. She proved to be an excellent subject and went into a deep trance in the first session. She was permitted to talk at will and began at once to recount a nightmare that she had had the night before, of the sort that constituted one of her presenting complaints. This was the beginning of a course of treatment in which the patient was seen every day for an hour to an hour and a half, six days a week for sixty-seven interviews. At first the interviews were conducted chiefly by one of the authors, (M.B.), and later by the other, (M.G.). Both authors were always present. The interview was always begun with a short session in the hypnotist's office, in which the patient usually described how she had felt during the last twenty-four hours, frequently summarized what she had learned in the previous day's hypnotic session and occasionally advanced new ideas and formulations that had occurred to her since that session. If the patient had dreamed the night before, she usually related this dream in the preliminary interview. The patient was then taken into another room and hypnotized. After the first few hypnotic sessions she was very easily placed in hypnosis simply by the therapist's counting to ten. After the hypnotic session, a few words were occasionally exchanged about how the patient was feeling, she sometimes made some comments upon the material of the hypnotic hour, and the appointment was made for the following day. After the first hypnotic session, the patient remarked that to her surprise she was able to remember everything that had gone on in hypnosis. She was reminded that nothing to the contrary had been suggested and thereafter she continued to remember all the material of the hypnotic sessions except in a few instances where amnesia was specifically suggested and in a number of others where the forgotten material proved to have special dynamic significance.

The technique which was followed in the hypnotic sessions was in general one of directed associations. Usually the hour was begun by taking up the topic which, from her pre-hypnotic remarks, appeared to be uppermost in the patient's mind. This was discussed with her until some question was reached which she was unable to answer or to which her answer was unenlightening to the therapists. The formulation that was then most generally applied was: "I will count to a certain number and when I reach that number you will tell me the first thing that occurs to you in connection with so-and-so." Variations of this formula were also used. Sometimes the patient was told that a single word would occur, sometimes a picture. When it was particularly difficult to elicit material, she would sometimes be told that a number would occur to her which would indicate the number of letters in a word, and then these letters would be obtained in jumbled order. For example, she was once told that at the count of five, a number would occur to her which would be the number of letters in a word, which would help to answer the question under consideration. The number turned out to be four. The therapist then counted to five to get a letter, which was "m". The other letters obtained similarly were "o", "b", "w", and the four as re-arranged by the patient spelled "womb". It would frequently take the patient some little time to recognize the word which was constituted by a jumble of letters, even when it was obvious to the therapists. Frequently we would ask the patient to associate to a certain idea by producing an earlier memory which had the same emotional connotations as the idea. These same types of associative techniques were used in the exploration of dreams. We found that the dreams as given in the hypnotic state, in contrast to the pre-hypnotic interview, were much more replete with significant detail through which their meaning could be more quickly learned.

A few specialized hypnotic techniques were also used. On a number of occasions, the patient was told that she would have a dream in connection with a certain problem and this was almost always successful. On several occasions the patient was made in hypnosis to complete an incomplete dream action. In one dream, for example, she searched through an entire house, though she did not know what she was looking for. The last place in which she was going to look was the basement. But as she began to go down the stairs she awoke in terror. In the hypnotic hour she was made to go down into the basement and describe what she found. On one occasion the technique of induced regression to an earlier age was used with rather striking results. The patient was regressed to the age of five. We asked her where babies came from. She told us that babies were vomited up but refused to tell her theory as to how they were made. That night she had a dream which was a repetition of an experience at the age of five, in which she had been told of fellatio by a little girl friend. She then told us that it was this memory that she had refused to communicate while she was regressed.

The interviews were conducted with a great deal more activity on the part of the therapist than is the case in the usual psychoanalytic interview. The hypnotic interviews at times approximated question and answer interviews, rather than prolonged, uninterrupted, spontaneous verbalization on the part of the patient. The therapists followed whatever lead appeared to be the most promising and if after five or ten minutes it seemed to be yielding nothing, it was abandoned for another topic. Nevertheless, interpretations, except as will later be described with reference to transference phenomena, were kept at a minimum. Most interpretations were merely elaborations of the patient's spontaneous insight. Although it was the therapists' tentative formulations which led them to open certain topics, other psychiatrists who have read the verbatim records of the sessions have agreed that almost always the patient's formulations were spontaneous. This spontaneity was further attested to by the fact that much of the patient's production was unanticipated. The material unfolded with dramatic rapidity and withal in a well-ordered sequence. Most hours ended with unresolved problems and the patient frequently began the next hour by plunging into the previous day's problem as though the intervening twenty-four hours were blotted out.

Her freedom of behavior in hypnosis was in vivid contrast to that of the ordinary hypnotic subject as we usually see her in the experimental situation. At first she sat immobile, just as a subject usually does. But one day she moved her arm in describing something. She was startled to find that she had moved it, but when it was pointed out that she had not been prohibited from moving, her behavior became more and more free until soon there were hours when she was pounding on the arms of her chair in furious anger, and others in which she wept in despair, all the while in deep hypnosis. This illustrates what we believe to be one of the most important aspects of the treatment. Hypnosis can take place in a permissive atmosphere in which the patient can be given wide latitude of expression and behavior. Hypnosis can be divested of its time honored implications of the subject's absolute subservience, and immobility, and helplessness to act except under the initiation of the all-powerful hypnotizer.

When we were attempting to explore more adequately a memory that the patient had recalled, we would frequently suggest that the recall would be as vivid as though she were again experiencing the original event. The actions with which the patient accompanied some of her verbalizations attested to the vividness with which she was re-living experiences. When she recalled in hypnosis how she had in a dream searched for something in the sky, she raised her head and moved it as though searching on high, although her eyes remained closed. When she was asked to look into an open grave, which in the dream she had been afraid to do, she craned her head forward with such genuine apprehension and expectation that the effect was quite eerie. She was unaware of such bodily movements and expressed amazement when they were called to her attention. In her verbalization she would switch back and forth in a remarkable way from past to present tense, as though she was at one moment oriented in the present and at the next moment vividly re-living the past. We feel that this intricate interweaving of the past and present represented the re-integration of the repressed past into her conscious ego.

Some of the patient's symptoms disappeared in the manner that Freud described as occurring in cathartic abreaction, and it was in connection with these that the experiences of re-living were most vivid. A notable example was her fear of falling which disappeared soon after the beginning of the treatment, immediately after her recall and re-living in hypnosis with intense affect two childhood falling experiences. In one she fell from a high chair and in the second, she fell from a hammock at the age of seven. It is difficult to describe the vividness with which she cried in terror: "Save me, Dr. B., save me—I'm falling!" That this re-living in hypnosis is not simply a re-living of the original experience but rather a re-living that takes place in the frame of the present personality structure is clearly shown by her calling on the doctor to save her—and indeed it is likely that it is this very difference that permits the resolution of the conversion mechanisms.

Other symptoms disappeared only when their symptomatic meaning had become clear to the patient. The hand-trembling, for example, was not completely relieved until the very end of the treatment when the patient developed what seemed to us to be full insight into its symbolic meaning.

The case material and dynamics which were actually obtained we do not report here. We plan to publish them in detail, but believe that it is more appropriate here to discuss the method rather than the individual case. In brief, it can be said that we obtained the kind of material that is familiar to all psychoanalysts in the psychoanalysis of cases of hysteria. We learned, for example, that the patient's vomiting represented *both* a rejection of impregnation and a fantasy of delivery, *both* of which she unconsciously thought took place by mouth. Material substantiating the psychoanalytic discoveries concerning infantile psychosexual development appeared in unusually clear and abundant detail, not simply in terms of reconstruction on the basis of fantasies, but rather by way of direct recall of childhood memories and ideas. By the end of the treatment the patient had been entirely relieved of her symptoms, not only those of somatic conversion, but also the psychological disturbances, such as her anxiety and depression. Shortly after she returned home her youngest child became seriously ill, and although some of her anxiety returned, she weathered the storm very much better than she had previous similar episodes. This experience, however, has led her to feel that she needs a few more weeks of treatment and she plans to return.

We call the treatment we used "hypnoanalysis" because we believe it combines significant features of hypnosis and psychoanalysis. We should like to discuss how the present method resembles and how it differs from each of these.

One of the basic differences between this treatment and hypnosis as previously used and one of its essential similarities to psychoanalysis is the handling and the use of the transference. Undoubtedly the most significant addition to the technique of psychoanalysis that Freud made after abandoning the hypnotic method in favor of free association was the recognition and the interpretation of the transference. It is now well recognized that the transference phenomenon exists in every psychotherapeutic situation—indeed in every relation between physician and patient and in many other life situations. The unique contribution of psychoanalysis is the awareness of and interpretation to the patient of this transference. The patient's recognition of his enactment in the psychotherapeutic situation of his previously formed behavior patterns is one of the most important vehicles by which he obtains insight.

Psychoanalysis is no longer the only method that makes conscious use of transference. An attempt has been made by a few psychiatrists to carry over the technique into general psychotherapy and many psychoanalysts believe that when the unconscious mechanisms of the patient-therapist relation are thoroughly understood by the therapist, any method of psychotherapy can be made more effective.

Although the dynamics of the induction of hypnosis have only begun to be explored, there seems little doubt that there is an intimate relation between the induction of hypnosis and the transference between hypnotizer and subject. This is not to deny that other factors may be involved too. Perhaps the first clear formulation of this point of view was made by Ferenczi who differentiated between "mother" and "father" hypnosis. He believed that the force impelling the subject to accept hypnosis was in the first instance love, and in the second, fear. Ferenczi attributes cures through hypnosis to the persistence in the patient of this unconscious transference. In our patient, the ease of hypnotizablity varied with the state of transference. When she was in an angry, rebellious mood, the hypnosis was somewhat more difficult to induce and was not as deep. When she was in a state of positive transference, she went quickly to sleep, with a deep sigh of unmistakably erotic significance.

We are here not so concerned with the significance of transference in the induction of hypnosis as with the interpretation of the transference as it arose within the hypnotic interviews. That is to say, we made no attempt to interpret the transference by which the patient became hypnotized, but we did interpret the transference which developed in the psychotherapeutic relationship in a manner very similar to that in a psychoanalysis. The patient's transference in this case ran the gamut from warm expressions of affection under the influence of which her symptoms were markedly alleviated simply by her entrance into the therapists' office, to wild outbursts of rage, anger and jealousy. The initial interpretations of the transference were an exception to the general rule that interpretations were not given by the therapist until spontaneously suggested by the patient. After these first interpretations, however, with explanations to the patient of the nature of transference, she spontaneously expressed her insight into the changing aspects of the transference just as she did into the progressive unfolding of the psychodynamics of her neurosis. The specific details of the transference could be given only in the light of the complete treatment history and therefore only a few examples will be given here: The patient vomited instantly when she learned that the psychiatrist's wife had just had a baby. She spontaneously recognized that this vomiting was based on the same jealousy and wish to have a baby by a father figure that she had felt when her siblings were born. Under the influence of an oral theory of birth she had as a child reacted to their appearance by vomiting. There were several instances of unusual transference behavior arising from the fact that the patient was being treated by a man and a woman together. The most striking of these occurred early in the treatment when, at the end of an hour, the therapists left the room for a moment before terminating the hypnosis. When they returned to the room the patient had become

severely nauseated and disturbed and explained that she had
suddenly recalled an experience of over-hearing parental intercourse. The recall had evidently been stimulated by the
absence of the two therapists. On another occasion, during
the patient's induced regression to the age of five, one of the
therapists whispered a remark to the other and the patient
called out, "I hear Daddy and Mother whispering—they have
too many secrets!"

There is a fundamental opposition between the handling of
transference in earlier forms of hypnosis and hypnosis as we
used it. In hypnosis by direct suggestion the hypnotist strength-
ens and exploits this unconscious transference by investing
himself with mysticism and an aura of the super-natural.
That Freud's difficulties with cathartic hypnosis had much
to do with the fact that he had not yet developed the technique of interpretation of transference can be clearly seen in
the following remarks from his autobiography: "Increasing
experience had also given rise to two grave doubts in my mind
as to the use of hypnotism even as a means to catharsis. The
first was, that even the most brilliant results were liable to
be suddenly wiped away if my personal relation with the patient became disturbed . . . and one day, I had an experience
which showed me in the crudest light what I had long suspected. One of my most acquiescent patients woke up on
one occasion and threw her arms around my neck." Freud
is obviously speaking of negative and positive transference.
Recent work of Erickson and Kubie reports the utilization of
the transference relationship to achieve therapeutic results,
but the transference itself is not analyzed. In the case which
we report, the interpretation of the transference was, as in
psychoanalysis, a vehicle by which we led the patient to insight into her neurosis.

The objection that is most frequently raised to the use of
hypnosis as a psychotherapeutic tool is the statement that
the ego of the patient with its resistances and defenses is not
involved. In fact, it is said that while this is the very reason

that one has direct access to unconscious material, it also accounts for the fact that hypnotic cures are so frequently temporary. It is believed that the hypnotic technique obliterates the dynamic activity of the ego, that whatever insight is gained is not assimilated into the ego, and that therapy therefore effects no significant change in the ego. We believe that this objection to hypnosis arises not because hypnosis in its very nature obliterates the ego, but because of the way it is used even in cathartic hypnosis. The attempt of the therapist in that method is simply to elicit the traumatic experiences under the theory that their re-living will cause their harmful effect to disappear by abreaction. No attempt is made to help the patients integrate newly gained insight into their egos. That the abdication of the ego is not a necessary condition of the hypnotic state, we believe has been thoroughly demonstrated by much recent hypnotic work. Our patient showed strong resistances, both in and out of the hypnotic sessions. At one point in the treatment, in a phase of strong negative transference and shortly before the emergence of some especially traumatic material, she was on the verge of disrupting the treatment to seek surgical relief for her complaints. Once when she was told in the hypnotic hour that she would have a dream the following night, she kept herself awake all night to prevent herself from dreaming. In the induced regression, when she was asked how babies are made, she replied, "I won't tell you, even if you spank me," and indeed did not tell. On many other occasions she at first refused in hypnosis to communicate the material present in consciousness.

The types of formulation of insight that our patient made in the hypnotic state were no different from those in the prehypnotic interviews. In hypnosis she reacted to the revelations about herself with the same shame, chagrin, and attempt at denial that she showed in the waking interviews. For many days her entire waking life was preoccupied with thoughts and ideas of the preceding hypnotic session. As already mentioned, despite the fact that she was an excellent somnambule, she did not have amnesia for hypnotic interviews.

As is to be expected in a case of anxiety hysteria, the patient's defense was basically strong repression. Presumably the conversion symptoms represented the points where repression alone was not an adequate defense. There seems to be no doubt that the hypnotic state is somehow able to break through the defense of repression probably in a way related to the phenomenon of hypnotic hypermnesia. The patient would frequently say, as though groping for a memory or an idea: "I know it's in my mind, but I just can't get it." She recalled one day, for example, that when she was five years old she had fallen off a porch and had broken her arm—an episode that she had long forgotten. She felt that there was something more but could not bring it into consciousness. In the next hour she continued to search for the elusive recollection that was just beyond her reach until she was almost in a frenzy of impatience. Suddenly, with climactic force, it burst on her that she had thrown herself from the porch in order to gain her father's attention and had accidentally broken her arm. She felt there was still more and was not satisfied until she had recaptured the final link in the memory which was that she was trying to call her father away from her mother who was in childbirth in the house.

Sometimes she was very reluctant to attempt to pursue a certain topic and then we would insist that she would be able to recall it, employing the various devices of counting, searching for words, and so forth. We broke through the resistance then, not by interpretations of the reasons for her loss of memory, nor by attempts to reach the memory through uncovering successive layers of superimposed screen memories, but rather by asking for direct recall. That the recall was forthcoming we feel must be a function of the hypnotic state.

We think that in the hypnotic state the ego and the resistances can be temporarily suspended to gain repressed material and that then, within the hypnotic state, this material can be reintegrated into the ego. The patient's spontaneous shifting from past to present tense, which we previously described, can be viewed as a switching, first out of and then back into the current ego orientation. How it is that hypnosis enables more direct access to the unconscious and the repressed, we do not know. It may be that it is by way of the revival of past ego orientations in which the repression had not yet taken place. We speculate that an important factor permitting this revival of past ego orientations lies in the patient's partial assigning of responsibility for her feelings and verbalizations to the hypnotist. But this abdication of responsibility is a two-edged sword. It enables the repressed material to appear, but for purposes of therapy it must not be permitted to divorce the ego from the proceedings or else the assimilation into the personality of the newly gained insight will not take place. We believe that the analysis of the transference in hypnotic psychotherapy plays a particularly important role in establishing such ego-participation.

Psychiatrists in many places are seeking shortened forms of psychotherapy which will nevertheless be effective. Unfortunately these short forms most usually deal only with superficial matters and overlook many of the transference manifestations. We believe that in some types of cases this hypnoanalytic technique will enable more rapid uncovering and resolution of the deeper problems and more adequate dealing with the transference than short psychotherapy permits, but without sacrificing the advantage of brevity.

We make no sweeping claims for this method of treatment and indeed would like to stress our recognition that it can be properly evaluated only by constantly bearing in mind that we dealt with a case of hysteria. The chief mechanism in hysteria is repression and the hypnotic state seems to be peculiarly effective in counteracting that form of defense. Nevertheless, we believe that there is sufficient warrant to investigate this method in other neuroses and we believe that as a technique in the rational therapy of hysteria, it offers great promise.

Follow-up note: This patient's "plan to return" never materialized. After four months, she failed to respond to follow-up inquiries. We finally obtained information about her through the visit of a social worker two and a half years after the patient's discharge. Although she had suffered a return of some of her symptoms, and still wanted more treatment, she felt that she had been significantly helped by her therapy. Her family had undergone many difficulties and had had to move to another part of the country. Despite her symptoms, the patient was actively caring for her home and family.

Hypnotherapy for Mental Illness in the Aged[*]

Hysterical Psychosis in a 71-year-old Woman

by Margaret Brenman, Ph.D.,
and Robert P. Knight, M.D.

Certain departures from the traditional technique of hypnotherapy have been presented in a preceding paper (4). We shall here discuss a variation of the technique described as it was employed in the treatment of an hysterical psychosis in a seventy-one-year-old woman.

We report this case because we were unable to find in the literature another case where, in treating so old a person, hypnosis was used not simply for the suppression of symptoms but for the development of insight into their meaning. We shall describe the evolution of the treatment, which began with the modest aim of alleviating by direct suggestion the patient's most prominent symptoms. This procedure was gradually replaced by one that elicited from the patient a progressive translation of the symbolic significance of her bizarre and violent symptoms, until after seventy hours of treatment she was symptom-free and well adjusted to her environment, and felt that she understood the "meaning" of her illness.

Presenting Illness

Six months after her husband's death which occurred one year before her admission the patient had begun to complain of acute stomach distress and resulting insomnia. Although she had been complaining for forty years of "gas on the stomach", which had begun during her sole pregnancy, it had never before so intensely disturbed her. A thorough clinical examination failed to reveal sufficient organic basis for her difficulties. As she became increasingly distressed, she was per-

[*] Reprinted from: *The Bulletin of the Menninger Clinic*, 7:188-198, Sept.-Nov., 1943.

suaded to accompany her brother to his ranch. Here she became markedly depressed, complained incessantly, and began
to avoid people. Gradually she began to talk of burning sensations throughout her body, of worms crawling in her extremities, and of the impending loss of her eyesight, her hearing,
and her mind. She then developed a tremor of her lower jaw
which soon developed into a series of generalized bizarre
"shaking spells". During these, she manifested all kinds of
strange and violent contortions, to be described, which she
declared she could not control and explained as the result of
the "gathering of that gas inside of me"; these contortions
would sometimes subside after she was successful in belching.
When the patient began to express suicidal ideas and fears
that she might hurt someone, her brother became alarmed and
brought her to the Sanitarium.

Historical Sketch

According to information obtained from her brother, the
patient was one of thirteen children; the family was closely
knit, and she had made relatively few friends but had at-
tracted many beaus in her girlhood. She had given piano les-
sons and taught school, and at twenty-eight had married a
quiet, withdrawn man who strongly disliked the city and so
had chosen a profession which necessitated his living in the
country. Because the patient could not tolerate country life
they lived separately during much of their married life, although they saw each other frequently. Whenever her husband was ill the patient always went to take care of him.

When she was about fifty, the patient found that he had
been surreptitiously giving money to a widow. Impulsively,
she went to see a lawyer for advice on a divorce action. Her
daughter believes that her father never forgave the patient
this impulse, even though she abandoned it almost immediately; the daughter believes also that there were no real grounds
for so drastic an action and maintains that although the widow
had pursued her father, the relationship had never really de-

veloped. During the last three years of her husband's life, the patient lived with him on a farm, ministering to his needs.

Reactions to Hospital Care

When the patient was brought to the Sanitarium she kept up an incessant stream of plaintive remarks which detailed what appeared to be an almost delusional view of her symptoms. She repeated frequently that she needed a "stomach specialist" and resisted with violent emotional outbursts any attempt to discover existing psychological difficulties. She apparently felt she had been tricked into coming to a place where she would be "disposed of" and "used for research, but not treated". She seemed inaccessible, and her behavior was clinically pyschotic.

During her first two weeks at the hospital, the bizarre character of her behavior became more marked. The following account was written by her admitting physician:

"She spends the major part of her time in her room where she either sits quietly with an occasional rhythmic tremor of one leg or she paces back and forth hurriedly in her stockinged feet because she likes the feel of the cold floor. She writes lengthy letters to her sisters and daughter in which she describes her subjective reactions from moment to moment throughout the day as well as observations about other patients. Her bizarre movements usually increase markedly in the presence of the physician, nurses or other patients. The rhythmic tremors usually start in one extremity and increase rapidly in amplitude until all the extremities are involved; sometimes if the examiner restrains one extremity at the start, the rhythmic movement will appear elsewhere. During the physical examination the patient began to rub her abdomen rhythmically to demonstrate the presence of "the gas" and soon her whole body was involved in rhythmic convulsive-like movements. She shakes her wrists vigorously, stands with her hands on the bedstead, and then hops up and down with both feet while at other times she hops, almost leaps, about the room for a few moments while continuing to talk about herself. After these strenuous exertions she does not appear unduly fatigued. She frequently demonstrates the various movements to the examiner, while discussing them, in addition to displaying those which she says she cannot control. At times she emits resounding belches with seemingly great effort, pressing her abdomen during the process. She eats well and complains of still being hungry although she has hesitated to ask for re-orders. Several times she has slept with only a thin sheet over her during cold nights because she has felt so warm. While on walks she tries to leave her coat open. She objected strenuously to sedative packs and became almost resistive, bruising a toe as a result of her contortions while in a pack one day."

When the patient was discussed by the staff, it was unanimously felt that she presented not only an extremely difficult diagnostic problem but also a serious problem in institutional management. Treatment recommendations were exceedingly difficult to make, by reason not only of the atypicality of the syndrome but also of the complete inaccessibility of this patient. Because of the hysterical features in the clinical picture, the suggestion was given that an attempt be made to hypnotize the patient; it was hoped that additional anamnestic material might thus be elicited, and that a temporary alleviation of her most disturbing symptoms might be effected by direct suggestion. It was concluded that eventually electroshock treatment would probably be necessary. The prognosis was decidedly guarded.

Course of Hypnotherapy

The patient agreed, though reluctantly, to come for a trial session. She walked hesitantly into the room, glanced dourly at the therapist, and immediately fixed her hands on the desk, hopping violently on both feet, her teeth set and lips drawn back in a frenzy of exertion. When she momentarily ceased her hopping, she began to pat the desk-top with her hands in such a way that it appeared as though her hands were hopping over the desk. Suddenly she gave this up, left the desk, and strode with great energy back and forth, complaining loudly of the heat and smallness of the room and the absurdity of the type of care provided for her. She turned abruptly each time and finally stopped short, only to begin hopping anew, first on one foot and then on the other. Then she began to flail her left arm and to fan the air with her right hand at an incredibly rapid tempo. She finally sat down, on request, and when she was asked if it were possible for her to control these acts, she replied by holding her arms quietly on the chair; at this moment her right leg fairly leaped into the air and then began to pound the floor like a piston.

She tried to explain that her strange behavior fell roughly into two general categories: first, the kind of performance she was displaying at that moment, which she said was entirely beyond conscious control; and secondly, a type of "monkey-shines" which she thought she could possibly control, but felt she "had to do". To illustrate this second type of behavior she described a ritual which she had gone through hundreds of times at her brother's ranch. She would hold a handkerchief aloft, let it drop, and then watch to see whether "it stood up straight in a point" or whether "it just fell flat". Another example consisted of her getting down on all fours in the train compartment and "rearing around like a dog", much to her brother's consternation.

The results of the first few attempts to hypnotize the patient were extremely discouraging. She made no attempt to conceal her deep scorn for the procedure and, at first, would not cooperate even to the extent of sitting down for more than two consecutive minutes. She would suddenly jump up, shouting, "I can't concentrate", and commence to hop and whirl around the room. Typical of her derisive remarks was: "It would be better to take an enema than to come down here." When such remarks were countered with a friendly and slightly cajoling attitude, she would seem temporarily ashamed and make an

obvious effort to cooperate with the barest mechanics necessary for the induction of hypnosis.

Gradually the patient's attitude changed from frank resistance to a reluctant, perfunctory acquiescence to the request
that she sit down or that she relax her body. This made possible a light hypnosis in which the direct suggestions were
made that she sleep better, that her violent contortions subside, and that her acute stomach distress be relieved. It soon
became apparent that these suggestions were taking effect, inasmuch as her hyperkinetic movements had markedly decreased.[1] After six hypnotic sessions—over a period of two
weeks—the patient grudgingly admitted that she was improved,
but she maintained firmly that this was to be attributed to
excessive sedation and that now we were turning her into a
"dope fiend"; she thought she would ask to have the treatments discontinued.

It was not until the twelfth hour that a clear-cut turning
point in the treatment occurred. Hitherto very little attempt
had been made to convince her of the difference between the
normal and the hypnotic state; it had been her tacit assumption that she had been "going along" with the treatment because her daughter wanted her to, but that she had not been
responding in any way. During this hour, however, it was
apparent to the therapist that she was in a deeper state of
hypnosis than ever before. Accordingly, she was told she was
unable to open her eyes. She laughed, said, "Nonsense", and
proceeded to try. When she found to her amazement that she
could not, she smiled in some embarrassment, saying, "You
really have got the best of me, haven't you?" At the conclusion
of this hour, she asked if she might be scheduled for several
additional appointments each week, and from this time on
her attitude was eager, friendly and completely cooperative.
Because of this remarkable shift in her attitude, we decided to

---

[1] This subsidence of her motor symptoms was progressive and gradual during
the remaining period of treatment. They were completely absent when she left
the Sanitarium.

abandon direct suggestion for a more dynamic procedure which would provide the possibility of her gaining some insight into the significance of her illness. We did not expect to elicit any dramatically illuminating material, and certainly did not hope to gain a real understanding of the symbolic significance of her symptoms. We hoped only to help her to verbalize a portion of the emotional conflicts which she might regard as precipitating factors. She had hitherto obstinately refused to discuss any personal matters. The specific techniques used were generally similar[2] to those described in a previous report (4).

We were startled a day later when, during the hypnotic session, the patient began to talk with extraordinary freedom. She was asked in hypnosis to "go back" to the time when her insomnia first began and to speak aloud whatever occurred to her. She said:

"I hear Ed . . . going down the front steps and oh . . . it's awful, awful . . . wicked, selfish . . . I am thinking . . . of, could I have ever really thought that . . . yes, I know I did . . . I'm thinking I wish he were dead!"

She spent the remainder of the hour elaborating this theme, interrupting herself to sob bitterly over the memory of the hostility which had characterized the twenty years since she had suspected her husband of infidelity and had consulted a divorce lawyer.

During the next few hours, she continued to express with great emotion the almost irreconcilable opposites of her feeling toward her husband. She had admired and respected him, and thought of him as "a prince among men", but she had wanted him to love her in a warm and demonstrative manner, and had hated him for his coldness. Apparently he could never show any real affection, even before her impulsive trip to the lawyer. Throughout it was extremely difficult to assay the

---

[2] One practical difference lay in the fact that in this case only one author (M. B.) had actual contact with the patient. The progress of the case was, however, followed in minute detail by the other author (R. P. K.) and was supervised by him.

character of the patient's husband, but the available data suggested that he was an extremely schizoid individual who never
became genuinely intimate with anyone and who, after he
became impotent in his fifties, indulged in a kind of genteel
Don Juanism. This took the form of helping attractive middle-
aged widows who were in financial distress. The patient spoke
with great bitterness of these episodes and felt during the last
years of his life that she could not tolerate the "grudge" she
carried toward him for rejecting her; she thought that when
he died it "would be all over" and that she would be relieved
of her burden of frustration and hate. She had felt, too, that if
he died he would no longer be able to "carry on" with other
women and that again she would be "first in his life".

Her first effort to translate her symptoms into meaningful
terms came in answer to the direct question: "What are you
trying to express by these different acts?" She replied on two
separate occasions that they were a "release" and a "satisfaction", but was still unable to say what she meant by these
terms. She provided a clue, however, by following this response with a criticism of her hospital physician who had
made her "speechless with rage" when he had attempted during the preliminary history taking to question her about her
"sacred relationships" with her husband.

As she was discussing what she termed her "agitation", she
suddenly had a vivid visual impression of her husband seated
at a table, but added, almost sorrowfully: "I can't say that I
see the food." Actually the patient's appetite had gradually
increased since the onset of her illness, and she frequently
mentioned this as a saving grace; she wrote to her daughter:
"I am so *very, very* hungry; I eat up every crumb from my
tray. Must be the medicine they give me." This preoccupation
with food and eating, with hints of food deprivation, suggested a symbolic significance and this was confirmed in the
succeeding discussion of her "nervous indigestion".

She regularly gave associations of a frankly sexual content
in answering her own question, "What caused my gas?" but

thought them "silly" and "irrelevant" until the consistency of their appearance brought her to the realization that she regularly linked her adolescent and adult conflicts regarding genital sexuality with her alimentary disturbances. She spontaneously offered the information that "the sex part of my marriage never nauseated me at all", but shortly thereafter described herself as having felt "trapped" into becoming pregnant, and it was during this pregnancy that her chronic gastrointestinal difficulties had begun. She had acceded to her husband's demand for a child, hoping thus to "win his favor", after he had bitterly commented that a childless wife was no better than a prostitute. The patient devoted almost ten hours to this problem and gradually gave up what had been previously a tedious barrage of whining complaints about "this terrible gas gathering inside of me".

For a brief period following the discussion of this problem, the patient was aware of an intense sexual interest in several of the male patients. This development shocked and alarmed her; but after she had been assured that these feelings would not continue at such a pitch, she settled down to a kind of flirtatiousness which is socially acceptable in elderly ladies.

The patient now attacked the problem of translating the symbolism in what she termed her "monkeyshines". She was told in hypnosis to re-experience her feelings and thoughts in relation to the described handkerchief ritual. At first, she replied simply:

"Win or lose . . . win or lose . . . I see . . . if it stands up in a peak, I win; if it falls flat, I lose."

She added then that this made no sense whatever. During the next several hours, she extended the introspections accompanying the ritual. She suddenly felt the behavior was somehow related to her husband, and finally said:

"It meant if it stood up, I could entertain a thought that we could be friends again and if it fell down flat,

my hopes were in vain. But that was so foolish, because he was already dead."

When she was asked why she chose this specific act, she
could not say. The technique of inducing vivid visual experiences was now introduced; the patient was told that she would
see an object as though it were projected on a screen and that
the image would be the object which the handkerchief symbolized. At first, she stalled ingeniously by saying that she
could see an object dimly but that it was behind the screen
and so was obscured. Gradually she began to see shifting out-
lines, the clearest of which was "the huge strong body of an
elephant—his strong limbs"; this was quickly followed by the
image of an "extremely beautiful woman" in a glamorous pose.

Shortly after this experience she volunteered the following:

> "You know—I have been telling you that when my
> husband lost his desire I lost mine too—and that it
> didn't matter to me a bit . . . In fact it seemed to me
> that I didn't even miss that sacred relationship, but
> yesterday it suddenly flashed into my mind that for
> years and years I kept dreaming about having that
> sacred relationship with Ed . . . In my dream I would
> think to myself, 'At last I've done it—at last it's hap-
> pened. Now we will be friends again!' Not that the
> sacred relationship is all there is to marriage but it
> seemed like if I could get him to become interested
> in me again that way that perhaps we could start all
> over again."

Directly following this statement the patient was asked
whether all of this had anything to do with the handkerchief
ritual. She laughed embarrassedly, blushed, and asked whether
the handkerchief might have symbolized her husband's "organ".
At the close of this hour she said, "That hour was a real satisfaction to me somehow. I don't understand why, but I feel
different than when I came."

Now it appeared that this insight released a flood of associations, all of which pointed to a formulation that her grotesque

bits of behavior had been a symbolic "acting out" of her deep need to undo the long estrangement from her husband by renewing their sexual relationships. Although it is not possible in the available space to detail the gradual unfolding of these, a few of the patient's conclusions will be mentioned. She recalled, for example, that directly following her husband's death she had been seized by an uncontrollable desire "to lie down on my back in bed". To explain her "rearing around like a dog", she suggested the fact that "animals have no restrictions". The patient interpreted her "hopping spells" in the following way:

> "Well, it seems if a person were happy they might be hopping up and down with joy . . . Maybe my subconscious was saying, 'Ed and I are friends again . . . isn't it wonderful . . . now we're together again, now it's all solved' . . . but that seems more like a little child would express being happy . . . Seems like when I was a little girl if something very nice were going to happen, I would hop up and down or jump all around the room."

During the final ten hours of her treatment, the patient seemed eager to make intelligible each detail of her bizarre behavior. It was as if a key to a code had been given, and she were simply applying it to the deciphering of dozens of specific messages. She stated that the repeated patting of coverlets and desks symbolized an attempt to reinstate her old way of "getting Ed ready", and that her fanning movements were an attempt to cool herself down. She said she had felt like "a dog in heat", and thus explained her terrible burning sensations.

It would appear that the patient's illness was a fantastic attempt to solve the long-existing problem of her relationship with her husband by a series of symbolic actions. She summarized it by saying: "Seems like what I was trying to do all along was to become friends with Ed—and it seemed that the way to become friendly was to start having relations with him again." No mention has been made of the aggressive aspects of the patient's symptoms; it seemed throughout that these were quite secondary to the erotic gratification which her symptoms provided. However, it should be pointed out that many of her symptoms had a "restitution value"—to undo her death wishes against her husband, bring him back to life, and reinstate a good relationship between them.

Discussion

Even after seventy hours of intensive treatment, it was not possible to place this patient in any one of the standard diagnostic categories. On admission, and for several weeks thereafter, she was clinically psychotic. Despite her advanced age, she showed no significant senile symptoms. She exhibited some features of agitated depression and even some paranoid elements in her suspiciousness and in her delusional view of her somatic symptoms. However, these were overshadowed by the long-standing organ-neurosis, focused on gastrointestinal difficulties, and by her compulsive rituals[3] and hyperkinetic movements. The last mentioned symptoms often gave witnesses the impression of being relatively close to conscious control and thus were reacted to by her relatives with some irritation, as though she were consciously "faking". This reaction, so frequently elicited by hysterics, together with the remarkable recovery of memories dating back fifty and sixty years, speak for a diagnosis of hysteria. However, inasmuch as her behavior went beyond the recognized limits of a neurosis, we were led to apply the almost obsolete diagnostic term "hysterical psychosis" because it most nearly described her unusual syndrome.

The highly symbolic motor expression of her unconscious strivings raises a provocative theoretical problem. We know that in the normal individual unconscious wishes are constantly trying to "force their way through the pre-conscious system

[3] Insofar as the patient perceived her repetitive bizarre behavior as ego-alien and beyond conscious control, such behavior might be thought of as "compulsive". However, the fact that these acts afforded her frank gratification renders questionable the use of the term "compulsive".

to consciousness and the command of motility" (1); the powerful counterforces relax only at night and permit some of these
impulses entrance into consciousness, but even then this freedom is limited by the fact that the impulses are heavily disguised
and the "gate to motility" is closed. Freud, speaking of the
action of unconscious wishes in sleep, says:

"No matter what impulses from the usually inhibited unconsciousness may bustle about the stage, there is no need to
interfere with them; they remain harmless, because they are
not in a position to set in motion the motor apparatus which
alone can produce any change in the outer world" (1).

He points out, moreover, that in two conditions this "safe"
relationship of unconscious wish and available motility does not
exist: in psychoses and in somnambulism (1) (2). He says psychosis may occur under two conditions: when there is a "pathological enfeeblement of the critical censorship" or a "pathological reinforcement of the unconscious excitations", either of
which may bring about the condition in which "forbidden"
unconscious impulses and potential motor expression exist
simultaneously. He feels that we do not know what conditions
the phenomenon of somnambulism, and wonders why it does
not occur more frequently. No answer has been suggested
by subsequent research and the problem stands substantially
as challenging as it was when Freud called attention to it.
One can do little more than to point to additional questions.

At the center of these seems to stand the still obscure relationship between unconscious wishes and available motility.
We know certain of the phenomena that presumably emerge
from different variations of this relationship, but we know
nothing of the specific factors that produce each. For example, we know that in certain psychoses the motor apparatus
provides the means of expression of undisguised impulses,
normally unconscious, as for example the carrying out of mur-
der, rape, or arson. Yet, in others, as in the present case, unconscious impulses are given motor expression but are so heavily disguised that the original impulse cannot be discovered

except by the application of specialized techniques of psychological investigation. Fundamentally the same problem arises in any attempt to understand the acting out of dreams in somnambules. It might be that all of these apparently disparate phenomena can be made more intelligible if they are studied with reference to Freud's original formulations regarding the normal relationships of unconscious impulses and "gates to motility" in the waking life and in sleep.

We come now to a discussion of the treatment technique. In a previous paper (4) there were described the essential differences between a dynamic hypnotherapy and a technique that employs hypnosis to the end of directly suggesting the suppression of symptoms; both of these methods of treatment were compared with psychoanalysis, and it was concluded that it may be possible to combine hypnotic and psychoanalytic techniques in such a way as to shorten the period of treatment without sacrificing the insight usually necessary for a permanent recovery. In that paper especial emphasis was laid on the appearance of transference phenomena and the insight derived from these phenomena and their interpretation.

In the present case, no significant transference phenomena—in the psychoanalytic sense—were manifest during the course of treatment. Beyond the special kind of "transference" that underlies any successful hypnosis, the patient's personal attitudes toward the therapist were restricted to normal respect, confidence, and cooperation. Moreover, very little material from her childhood was discussed with the patient. Her occasional attempts to revive these memories in detail were not encouraged; a resolution of acute current problems was the most we believed should be attempted at her advanced age.

A survey of the cases successfully treated by hypnotherapy in our experience shows that significant variations in technique have been employed in various types of patients. The only common elements are the production of the trance and a more productive working together of patient and therapist than exists in other types of psychotherapy. Hence one would be led to suggest that hypnotherapy is distinguished from psychotherapy mainly by the effect of the hypnotic trance in lessening the ego resistance. It appears that such resistance can largely be circumvented by hypnosis, making it possible to eliminate side-issues and thus to shorten considerably the time required for treatment. The hypnotic technique in the present instance made accessible a patient who was entirely inaccessible to any other kind of psychological approach. It made possible the recovery of directly relevant memories, the tentative formulations by both patient and therapist, and the ultimate necessary insight.

Thus it appears that hypnotherapy can accent any of the elements that may be accented in various kinds of psychotherapy. Among these are: direct suggestion, reassurance, the recovery of memories and "abreaction", and transference phenomena, with recall and insight dependent on and derived from these phenomena. The latter are more specifically psychoanalytic and should perhaps be manifestly utilized therapeutically in order that a hypnotherapy be considered "hypnoanalysis".

The particular choice of these factors must be adapted to the individual case. Thus the only requisite for hypnotherapy is that the patient be hypnotizable, and the only common factor in divergent applications of hypnosis is the circumvention of ego resistances via the hypnotic trance.

Summary

The case of a seventy-one-year-old woman with an "hysterical psychosis", treated successfully by hypnotherapy in seventy hours, is presented. The special features of the case are the advanced age of the patient, the bizarre nature of the symptom picture, the inaccessibility to other attempts at therapy, and the rapid recovery with insight through hypnotherapy.

Diagnostic problems of the case are discussed and special attention is directed to the modifiable hypnotherapeutic technique, particularly as it differed from a previously reported case in which outstanding transference phenomena made possible employment of a combined hypnotic and psychoanalytic technique.

Follow-up note: This patient continued well for two years after discharge. Without any apparent precipitating event, she developed a severe depression and was rehospitalized. Features of senile change were evident but their role was difficult to evaluate. She did not respond to "expressive" hypnotherapy as before (though she was still hypnotized) and finally shock treatment was used with hypnosis as a supportive adjuvant to the psychotherapy which followed. For the past four months she has again been making an independent extramural adjustment but on a significantly lower level than before.

Techniques of Hypnoanalysis, a Case Report[*]

BY MERTON M. GILL, M.D.,
AND KARL MENNINGER, M.D.

This paper issues from the research on the combined use of hypnotic and psychoanalytic techniques being conducted at the Menninger Clinic. It will describe the hypnoanalytic treatment of a patient presenting a varied symptomatology, including neurasthenic, hysterical and depressive features. Our major emphasis will be on material illustrative of the technique, although we shall also discuss some more general aspects.

The Case History

The patient was a thirty-six-year-old housewife, married to a moderately successful professional man living in a small southern town. When asked to give her chief complaint she stated: "I didn't come here because I thought I needed to; I came because the doctor said I was psychoneurotic and my husband agreed with him and asked me to come. If he had told me I had to come, I wouldn't have come, but I came only to please him."

In spite of this, the patient gave a long story of somatic complaints and illnesses extending back over many years. When given an opportunity, she launched into a description of these, beginning with a cold at the age of two weeks and a boil at the age of one month and ending with the present complaints of headaches, diarrhea, cardiac palpitation, excessive sweating, depression and "nervousness" and frequent disturbing dreams. The patient had had several repairs of the cervix uteri, two Caesarian sections, an appendectomy, and an ovarian operation. In 1941 she had been hospitalized for a year at a tuberculosis sanitarium with a diagnosis of bronchiectasis. When

[*]Reprinted from: The Bulletin of the Menninger Clinic, 10:110-126, July, 1946.

informed by us that the physical examination revealed no significant organic disease, she was resentful and expressed the view that our studies had been incomplete.

Despite these and other evidences of antagonism and resistance, such as her refusal at first to complete the psychological tests because they took longer than she had anticipated, the patient responded rather quickly to a sympathetic attitude, completed the diagnostic study and accepted the treatment recommendations.

According to the history given by her, she had been reared in a small New England community. Her father, though a man of very modest means, held a respected position in the community and was a pillar of the church. He was always "nervous" and easily upset. He died several days after a fall at the age of sixty-seven, having been nursed in this last illness by the patient. The patient's mother, described as warm and devoted to her children, was living and well at the age of sixty-five. The patient was the fourth of eight siblings of whom only four are still living. The only one who figured prominently in the treatment was a three-year-younger brother. The history seemed to indicate clearly a turning point in the patient's life at about the age of thirteen. She was severely ill then with typhoid fever and an older sister who contracted it at the same time died of it. During convalescence from this fever the patient developed many presumably functional disturbances including tremors, smothering spells and episodes of anorexia. The doctor advised her "to live as though she had tuberculosis" and as a result the patient's high school career was marked by an avoidance of the usual extracurricular and social activities with strong emphasis on doing well in her studies. She was thus set off from her school-mates as separate and "queer". She taught school from seventeen to nineteen, then had two years of college followed by a year of work after which she married. She had three pregnancies, two, six and eight years respectively after marriage. All of these were turbulent. The first baby, a boy, lived only two hours and his death was ascribed to a birth injury during the difficult labor. The last two were also boys, both delivered by Caesarian section, the first of them living and well at the age of eight but the second dead (at birth) of some congenital defect of the lungs.

Three months after the birth (and death) of this child, the patient suffered a "nervous collapse" ascribed to her depleted physical condition, grief over the loss of her child, and the "unreasonable" demands of a women's club to which she belonged. The collapse was characterized by insomnia, marked increase of tremor in her hands, irritability and restlessness, together with a special fear of sharp instruments, with the feeling that if she were not prevented from doing so she would seize a knife or scissors and plunge it into her heart. The many physical difficulties described at the time the patient presented herself at the Clinic were present at this time also and continued then for the next six years—i.e., up to the time of her admission to the Clinic—in spite of much medical therapy.

The psychiatric examination revealed a small, neatly dressed woman who, despite her expressions of resentment against doctors, her protestations that she was being unjustly stigmatized as psychoneurotic, and her sometimes tedious insistence on detailing her multiple somatic complaints, gave the impression of being a basically friendly and warm person. She showed marked anxiety, many nervous mannerisms, and a marked fluctuation of mood, though with a keynote of depression. Her thought processes were intact. A diagnosis of psychoneurosis with neurasthenic, hysterical and depressive features was made, with the probability that at least some of the somatic complaints were conversion phenomena. These findings were confirmed by the psychological tests which pointed in addition to much inhibition about sexual matters and to the possible presence of some obsessive ideation.

Hypnotizability Study

During the preliminary examinations the patient was studied for hypnotizability. At first the indications were rather disappointing, only a slight hypnosis being obtainable. An attempt was then made to deepen the hypnosis with intravenous sodium pentothal; the technique used was to inject the pentothal and carry out the same hypnotizability test with the suggestion that the effect achieved by the drug could be produced without it, thereafter. Under the pentothal, hypnotizability was slightly improved but (in the next test) without pentothal, it was much improved with partial immediate and posthypnotic amnesia and the patient was accepted for hypnoanalysis.[1] A formal re-test of hypnotizability was not carried out until the treatment was well advanced and then it was found that the patient was capable of deep hypnosis with complete amnesia and, as will be later described, a regression to an earlier age could also be accomplished.

General Description of the Treatment Technique

The patient was seen in fifty-minute interviews, five times a week for a total of 133 interviews. Almost without exception these were conducted with the patient in the hypnotic state. She would come in, lie down, listen to the therapist's count to ten, lapse into deep hypnosis, and begin talking. The therapist sat in view of the patient, not behind her, but throughout the interview her eyes would be closed, since a sleeping type of hypnosis was induced from the beginning with the suggestion that the patient would be unable to open her eyes. Hypnosis was terminated by saying the letters from A to G and marked by the opening of her eyes. She would then arise and leave promptly except upon a few occasions when she was slightly dizzy after a hypnotic regression. The patient spontaneously reported dreams almost from the start, and for the first ten hours an attempt was made to deal actively with these with the hope of reaching interpretations at once. When it became clear that this was doing little other than to stimulate the patient's resistance, the technique of free association was explained and thereafter it was understood that the patient was

---

[1] Numerous attempts to repeat this improvement of hypnotizability through the use of pentothal with other patients have been uniformly unsuccessful.

to associate freely unless the therapist actively intervened with an interpretation or some special instruction. This and other experiences have convinced us that this is the most fruitful and practical technique to use in the beginning of a hypnoanalytic treatment. Even later on, the technique of free association, unless the therapist otherwise intervenes, seems to be the best. During the period of therapy amnesia was produced temporarily for the material of one interview to test the depth of the hypnosis. Otherwise it was never suggested nor did it spontaneously develop; the patient always remembered the material of the hypnotic interviews.

The Material of the Interviews

Before describing some of the special hypnotic techniques employed, we will give a brief survey of the material which appeared during the course of the treatment. There was nothing unusual about this material in content. It was almost certainly no different from that which would have been elicited had this patient undergone a psychoanalysis. The features that differentiate it are the relative rapidity with which it came, and the absence of long periods of resistance and digression. We do not believe that in a psychoanalysis of equivalent length this amount of "deep" material would have been obtained.

Summarizing this material will of course make it seem much more "pat" and logically consecutive than was actually the case. The treatment material falls into several distinct periods. The first period occupied sixty hours. After an initial period of orientation in which the patient expressed some lack of confidence in the therapist because she was not sure of his religious principles, the first really important material was the confession of a platonic love affair in college. In fantasy there still persisted strong feeling for the man, though she now had almost no contact with him. After this confession there appeared a progressive concentration on her wish for father and therapist, culminating in a dream in which the patient seemingly was thirteen years old, and was rejected by her father. This was correlated with the recollection that at the age of thirteen she had pressed herself against her father in an embrace, had felt his penis against her body and had become sexually aroused, was pushed back by him and sternly told never to do that again. It was this episode which had accounted for the turning point in the patient's life at the age of thirteen which had seemed so clear in the history. Following this memory, all the patient's symptoms dramatically disappeared and she wanted to conclude the treatment and go home. She was told she was making excellent progress but that if her recovery was to be lasting more work would have to be done. She reluctantly agreed to stay and almost at once many of the symptoms returned.

The next forty hours (61st to 100th) were concerned with progressively clearer expressions of feelings of inferiority, at first related to her small stature, her feeling of educational and intellectual inadequacy, then more clearly her repudiation of femininity and envy of masculinity, until finally she clearly recognized her penis envy. After this she said that "an internal pressure which I have felt for years has suddenly been released".

The third period (the 101st to 119th hours) dealt with her feeling that she had been cheated by God who had made her a girl, and with her long time hope that a penis would grow. In hypnotic regression it was found that she believed menstruation was caused by the monthly tearing of a small piece of flesh which might otherwise have grown into a penis. It also became clear that she hoped to get a penis from the therapist and was resentful and disappointed by his failure to give her one. This was followed by recognition of her unconscious wish to get the envied penis by forcibly taking it away from a man. In the 118th hour she reported a dream in which a man did something to her from behind and left his penis in her. In the dream she thought to herself, "this is what I wanted", but then changed her mind, took out the penis and threw it away.

In the last fourteen hours (120th to 133rd) there was gradually diminishing evidence of resentment that she could not have a sexual relationship with the therapist and also get a penis from him, terminating in a dream of a house (obviously her own body) which she had seen before in a run-down and inferior condition but which now seemed quite acceptable; she also dreamed that the therapist gave her a token of affection by kissing her and then saying goodbye. She seemed under a fair degree of pressure to return home, and left a few days earlier than she had at first planned so that she could attend a special meeting of her women's club.

At the close of the treatment the patient was free from all her symptoms with the exception of a slight tremor when in particularly disturbing situations. The mechanisms producing the somatic symptoms were only partially clear. The diarrhea ceased when the patient began to speak really freely with the confession of the affair in college. Headache regularly reappeared when an attempt was made to force the emergence of disturbing material. The excessive sweating gradually disappeared but its mechanism was not elucidated beyond its familiar association with anxiety. The fatigue disappeared as the problem of weakness and inferiority related to femininity was worked through. The only suggestions about the dynamics of the tremor were that it seemed to her perhaps the trembling of a weak feminine creature and it was perhaps related to a tremor which her father had had for many years and which the patient regarded as like her own.

In a follow-up letter several months after leaving treatment the patient reported that her breasts had been a little sore for several weeks and that first she and then her husband independently had noticed that they increased a little in size. The patient recalled that during adolescence she had tightly bound her breasts in the attempt to hide their development. During the treatment she had at times expressed the feeling that her breasts were not large enough. She herself interpreted this belated growth as resulting from the fuller acceptance of her femininity which the treatment had made possible.

Psychological tests were repeated during the patient's last week in treatment. The comparative report states that the previously existing depressive trends were no longer present. This was shown by the rise of the I.Q. from 108 to 126, the increase of the Rorschach responses from 14 to 21, and greater speed in the word-association test. The report further noted "greater freedom for the expression and experiencing of affect and anxiety. Association disturbances to words of sexual connotation were much less marked than in the first test".

A recent follow-up report two years after discharge stated that the patient is free of symptoms and leads a busy and happy life. A striking feature of the follow-up letters from the patient is the continued work she has attempted by way of analysis of dreams and other material. One of these dreams will be reported later. This independent self-analysis certainly presents a much different picture from that which is ordinarily given of the hypnotic subject as a passive automaton capable of no initiative or independent thought and bound forever to the hypnotist by an unverbalized and unresolved affective tie.

Transference Material

Much of the transference material has already been indicated by implication in the statement of the psychodynamics. After the short initial period of irritability which has been described, the patient quickly developed an exaggerated deference to and regard for the therapist. She often called him "Sir" and once even inadvertently substituted his name for God in her prayers. Though this attitude was pointed out upon a number of occasions, it was never radically changed. It was still her attitude when the treatment closed. There were a few short-lived outbursts of resentment in response to such things as the suggestion that the treatment continue after disappearance of symptoms at the close of the first sixty hours and the examiner's refusal to give her advice about some practical matters such as whether she should room with another patient. On occasions when her wish to have sexual contact with the therapist or to obtain a penis from him appeared most clearly, she would sometimes react to interpretations with the feeling that the therapist was laughing at her for presuming to think of herself on intimate terms with him. A topic which was for some time almost taboo in the treatment was the subject of religion. The patient believed that the therapist "scoffed" at her religious principles and regarded her belief in the efficacy of prayer as naive foolishness. No attempt was made to analyze the patient's religious attitude except in superficialities. She herself, however, recognized the connection between her ideas about her father and about God and explained that an adolescent period of refusal to attend church was due to anger that God had made her a woman.

In the 36th hour the patient confessed for the first time to masochistic fantasies she had had for many years in which men cruelly mistreated prostitutes, especially by techniques of stretching the vagina. This proved to be related to an experience at the age of four when she had seen her father's penis, considering it very large, and to memories of her mother talking of intercourse as an unhappy duty. Further material seemed to indicate that these masochistic fantasies were related to the hypnosis, too. For example, the patient felt during the first phase of the treatment that in hypnosis she was "in the power" of the hypnotist. She was much disturbed by reading in the newspaper of a woman who was charged with enslaving two other women through the use of hypnosis and while discussing this was seized by a mixture of fear and sexual excitement. On one occasion when the therapist said, "We'll try something new today", the patient instantly felt a spasm in her vagina. The elucidation of the relationship between these masochistic fantasies and the patient's reaction to the hypnosis did not affect her hypnotizability at all. It must be stated, however, that the topic was not extensively treated. The patient was as deeply hypnotizable at the end of the treatment as at the beginning. On the last day that she was seen she was for the first time hypnotized with her eyes open.

Six months after the termination of treatment the patient sent in an extraordinary letter in which, among other things, she stated that she realized that during treatment her original neurosis had been replaced by a "substitute neurosis", that her neurotic attachment to the therapist had not been fully resolved during the treatment but that now, beginning by way of a dream which she had herself analyzed, the problem was solved. Her method of procedure with this and other dreams was to lie down as she had in hypnosis, close her eyes and allow herself to freely associate and work on the dream elements "just as I used to do with you". This procedure undoubtedly involves some form of autohypnosis. The patient dreamed:

"My husband and I were staying at a place which was not our home. We seemed to have two rooms which had a connecting door. The second of the two rooms was quite small and it was my private room. My husband did not enter this room though he sat in the other room and looked into the smaller room and watched me. The light in this private room of mine would not burn but enough light came in from the other room so that I could see enough to comb my hair. I tried to make the light burn but I could not. I asked my husband to help me make it burn but he only answered that he could not make it burn for me and I felt in the dream he was not interested. Then I went to a big room which was like a gymnasium. The lights were not on there either but I thought, 'I cannot make the light in my room burn but I can make all these lights burn.' I went to the fuse box, put in a new fuse, and one by one the lights began to come on until they were all burning. I wondered why I could not make the one light burn."

The patient interpreted the dream as follows:

"The one light in a room which only I enter represents you. I think that because I was having the struggle with my emotions concerning you at the time I dreamed this dream. The little room which only I entered represents my mind. The door being open so that my husband could see in represents my discussing my problems with him so that he knew what was going on inside my mind. The fact that he did not seem interested in helping me make the light burn represents his recognition that this feeling I had for you was not a healthful one and needed to be overcome. I think my continuing to use the room to comb my hair represents my desire to keep the feelings I had toward you. But though I realized I could not make that one light burn I consoled myself with the thought that I could make others burn. I do not know for sure what this means. The only thing I can think of is the fact that I get much more notice from men now than I did during the years I was most ill. I do not mean by that that there is anything that is not acceptable to my husband as well as to me, but for a long time I was pretty well ignored by men. They were polite to me but that was all. I think the lack of notice was caused by the same thing I mentioned to you one time, namely that I felt badly all the time and looked distressed. Now I am happy. I can laugh and joke and have fun and every once in a while I chance to say something they apparently think is witty. My husband includes me in lots of things he formerly did not. And he seems to enjoy my being with him when other men are around. For instance, there may be two or three men in his office laughing and talking with him and he will ask me to come in, too. It has been a good many years since he did that, because I always felt bad and I guess I put pretty much of a damper on things. That is what I think that part of the dream meant, not that I could make men fall in love with me but that though there was one whom I could not even see, I was not unsuccessful with everyone. It is embarrassing for me to tell you that there were times when I wanted very much to have you be interested in me, and you were completely successful in maintaining a doctor-patient relationship, which of course was right. To tell you this dream at all has been embarrassing to me because of the significance in other dreams which we discussed of turning on a light." [In these dreams a burning light was identified by her as symbolic of an erect penis.] "I debated a long time about including this one but finally felt that I really should because it was a dream that stayed on my mind until I worked it out. I would not work on it for a long time, but I could not quit thinking about it until I did. This dream and interpreting it was useful to me for it made me realize the truth of how I had felt toward you and it made me face facts so that I did begin to realize that I had a neurotic attitude toward you. With the recognition and admission in my own mind I made the first step toward overcoming the difficulty."

The patient concludes her discussion of the resolution of the transference by saying: "The unreasonable desires toward you have left and there now remains only a normal feeling of gratitude and devotion. The feeling I now have is that which I can express freely to anyone with no sense of there being something I must hide."

Specialized Hypnotic Techniques.

1. *The use of dreams.* It will be recalled that one of the patient's original complaints was of frequent disturbing dreams. In addition to working with her spontaneous dreams, these two ways of "producing" dreams were used: one by suggestion that clarifying dreams would take place that night, and the other by suggestion that "dreams" would appear during the hypnotic sessions. Dreams were suggested when the material seemed to be digressing from the main theme, when a clearer statement of the theme was desired, and when an equivalent dream was wanted to help interpret a dream which either the patient or the therapist was having difficulty in understanding. The dreams obtained were handled, in addition to the usual techniques of association and interpretation, by forcing the recall of forgotten elements and by insisting on a clearer view of obscure details.

An example will be given of a dream suggested after a period in which there was a digression initiated by the therapist who wanted to know more about the patient's sensations during induction and in the hypnotic state. The patient was told that she would dream a dream that night which "would return us to the main theme". She reported in the next hour, the 51st, the following dream:

Her father is seen sitting in the living room on a chair. He has no clothes on. He is apparently ill, looks emaciated, but is laughing and talking. She is bathing him; she wants to avert her eyes from his body but cannot because she has to bathe him. This, she feels, makes it all right to look at him. He tells her to hurry because she has to go to church. She goes to church with a man whom she doesn't know but in whose company she takes great pleasure. She had hoped to get to church early to rehearse something but finds to her annoyance that there are already many people there. Something is wrong with the lighting in the church. She attempts to replace a fuse but is unable to do so.

Her associations to this dream seem to make it clear that it represented a sexual wish for her father and for the therapist. The matter of bathing her father refers to caring for him in his last illness when she saw his penis. The man whom she takes to church is the therapist. He has to go there because she feels that the therapist is not sufficiently religious, and to overcome the fact that he is a Jew. Her hopes to have the church empty and the difficulty with the lighting would provide an opportunity for sexual contact.

The patient had difficulty in understanding the above dream despite the fact that it was worked on for several hours and therefore the next device to be described—the suggestion of an equivalent dream—was used. The patient was told that she would have a dream that night that would express the same thoughts more clearly. The next day she reported two dreams, though she said she didn't see how they could be related to the dream of her father and the church.

She is marrying a "part Negro". She knows that she has been married before and that her name is X——. She likes her husband-to-be very much but doesn't want any of her friends to know about it. In the second dream she is again being married, this time to a man by the name of Dumbowski. This time, too, she knows she has been married before and so has he. Dumbowski is a south-European of some kind and gives the impression of being a large man even though he is not very tall. (Not until the next hour did the patient admit that in the dream she had intercourse with Mr. Dumbowski.)

The south-European part-Negro is easily recognizable as the therapist. The patient immediately associated to the fact that the man was large, though not tall, the idea that this was just the feeling she had about her father and when she nursed him in his last illness she was surprised to see how lean he was. This was a link to the bathing scene of the preceding dream. The frankly sexual character of the dream about Dumbowski was then clarified and made it possible for the patient to accept and understand the dream about father and the man whom she took to church as a (sexual) wish for father and therapist.

Next will be described a dream suggested during the hypnotic hour. The example chosen is a dream suggested to elucidate another dream. In the 108th hour the patient reported this dream:

"I go into a shoe store, see a hat, try it on, think of buying it and decide not to, buy something else and leave the store. I then look at my purchase slip and realize that I was charged for the hat even though I did not buy it. I am outraged."

She was asked to re-dream the dream in hypnosis and this time added to it that she did not return to the store but walked down the street, descended some stairs, and came to a place that was like a sunken garden.

Though the sexual symbolism of the dream is obvious, questions as to its meaning brought little response. (Incidentally this point is worth noting because it offers evidence contrary to the idea that in a good hypnotic subject symbols in dreams can be always readily interpreted.)

In the next hour it was suggested that the patient dream another dream which would express the same idea. She did, as follows:

"I am walking down the street and feel big and powerful like my younger brother (a husky six-footer). I come home, look in a mirror, and am disappointed to see myself as I am."
The hat and the sunken garden, then, are respectively her wish to be powerful and have a penis like her brother, and the reality that she is small and a woman. That she paid for a hat but did not get it indicates her hope to get a penis from the treatment, though of course this was not made any clearer in the equivalent dream than in the first.

We will now discuss several techniques of working with dreams that are possible in the hypnotic state in addition to the ones usually employed in the waking state.

First will be described forcing the recall of forgotten portions of the dream. A dream is often forgotten in part or in full because it was too illuminating, having too completely escaped distortion. Its recovery would therefore be especially useful. In the 38th hour the patient reported this dream:

"I go to a tourist camp with my husband. I seem to know that this camp is used for immoral purposes. I go into one of the cabins with my husband who asks me to undress. There is some difficulty in drawing one of the blinds and my husband says it doesn't matter. I undress and become sexually aroused but my husband leaves me unsatisfied."
The patient was sure there was another part of the dream which introduced it but had been unable to remember it. She was told that she would recall it at the count of ten and did so. She then remembered that *"as my husband and I come to the camp a man who seems to be a manager is drawing pictures on a blackboard before a group of people."* She thought these pictures might have been of nudes.

There was then introduced the next technique to be described, that of forcing a clearer statement of details of the dream. It was insisted that the patient "look at the drawings" and describe them and identify the artist. The patient described the picture drawn as one in the Thematic Apperception test, one of the tests given during the diagnostic study, and the man drawing the picture was the psychologist who administered the test. The picture was of several scantily-clad people. The patient had been unable to tell the psychologist any story about this picture and felt that he would deduce from this the fact that she was disturbed about sexual matters. The details of this forgotten part of the dream then made it much easier both to interpret the dream and to lead the patient inescapably to the fact that the dream represented the patient's view of the treatment situation which she had erotized and in which she had felt frustrated by the therapist.

Still another way of working with dreams was described in a previous paper from this Clinic (5). In that case the patient was told to finish in hypnosis an incomplete dream. This device was not used in this case.

2. *Regression.* Hypnotic regression techniques played a significant role in the last quarter of the treatment. Two ways in which regression was used will be described: first to reproduce the initial appearance of a symptom, and second to strengthen insight by reproducing a time at which ideas deduced from the material were consciously present in their original form.

Regression to reproduce the initial appearance of a symptom is illustrated by the following episode: several times during the treatment the patient had talked about a peculiar feeling in her face. It seemed to be growing and her face and lips felt very thick. In the 106th interview—by which time her penis-envy had been well understood—she again reported this feeling. All she could associate to it was that she believed it began during either her first or second pregnancy. The patient was regressed with the instruction to return to the first time this symptom had appeared. She went back to the fifth month of her first pregnancy and described the feeling as being present. The request to directly interpret the symptom was fruitless and she was told she would have a dream and did so as follows: the dream was apparently a memory.

"It takes place at the beginning of my first pregnancy. I am sitting in the living room at home, my husband comes in and takes me on his lap, pats my face and says: 'You may be little now but you will grow. The baby will grow and you will grow too.'"

Since the patient already understood the significance of being small was to her being without a penis, it was easy to infer that this feeling of growth relates to growing a penis. This interpretation was difficult for her to accept, however, and she obviously had no emotional conviction about it.

This conviction was produced by the second use of hypnotic regression to be described, a return to a time when the fantasy of growing a penis might have been conscious. Since there had been much evidence that the patient associated menstruation with a genital injury, she was regressed to her first menstrual period. She said that at first she thought the blood came from her kidneys but now she thinks some little piece of flesh had been torn and was bleeding. She had imagined that she might grow a "wetter" like boys have, but now the little piece of flesh which might have grown into one was torn. She remembers reading a story in which a princess was turned into a prince and hoping that a fairy would wave a magic wand over her and turn her into a boy. She remembered that she and her brother would go out on the back porch to urinate and she would stand up to emulate him. She would pretend that she was holding a penis in her hand. All these ideas were expressed spontaneously in approximately these words.

The patient had been regressed to her first menstruation eight hours earlier in the treatment. At this time too she had expressed the idea that something tore and bled, but she went no further. In the hours between the two regressions to her first menstrual period the idea of growing a penis had first been introduced. It may be then that it was this which allowed such material to emerge spontaneously in the second regression. It might of course be objected that this was the result of suggestion. The question cannot be answered other than by pointing to the internal unity of the material or by taking up the general problem of the validity of hypnotic regressions.

3. *Specific explorations.* As we have already reported in a previous paper (5) and as has also been clear in this one, the use of specialized hypnotic techniques implies a good deal more activity and direction of the treatment by the therapist than is usually the case in a psychoanalysis. One of the advantages that this possesses is that the therapist can direct the material by deciding which trend he wants to explore further, choosing an episode in the history in which this trend seems to come close to the surface and then pursuing this by one of the special hypnotic techniques. For example, after this patient's penis envy and disappointment that she did not grow one had been worked through it was decided that she needed to understand something of her castrative wish toward men. The episode six years before in which she had had to fight the feeling that she would stab herself seemed to mean that she was reacting with guilt for a castration wish and hence felt impelled to cut herself. The patient was regressed to this episode and it was found that her conscious thinking at that time was that she considered her illness was ruining the lives of people about her and she should therefore kill herself. It was suggested that she dream in the regression about the fear of knives and she dreamed as follows:

"A surgeon tells me, 'I will cut and cut and cut, so that you won't have to kill yourself.'"

This was the first of a series of suggested dreams in which the following sequence of ideas appeared: First the patient felt that her genitals were torn by childbirth, then she dreamed of harm coming to her son which she seemed powerless to prevent though she was willing to sacrifice herself for him, and then clearly castrative wishes against men appeared as seen finally in the dream which has already been mentioned in which a man did something to her from behind and left his penis in her. In one of the very last hours the patient, regressed to the age of eight, expressed the fantasy of cutting off her brother's penis with a pocket-knife and sticking it onto herself.

4. *Forcing associations and interpretations.* In this case we used for the first time a new technique for getting answers to questions in addition to those described in a previous paper. The patient was told that she would write on a blackboard in her mind and that she would not know what she was writing and would be unable to read it until it had been entirely written. On a number of occasions she would produce no associations to a dream or an idea when directly asked to do so, but relevant and revealing material could be obtained by use of this blackboard technique. Often she would have to be urged quite insistently before she would read what she had written. This technique is likely related to automatic writing. It is as though the material escapes censorship more easily because it is not recognized in consciousness while it is being produced. But because a record is made, in the case of automatic writing on paper and in this technique on an imaginary blackboard, this record can be presented to consciousness which must then face interpretation.

5. *Direct suggestion.* Hypnosis was occasionally used as a medium for direct suggestion for the temporary alleviation of symptoms. There were periods in the treatment when the patient's headaches were severely exacerbated, obviously in relation to disturbing material. Weekends, during which she had no treatment hours for two days, were often extremely difficult for her because of headaches. It was therefore occasionally suggested that she be free of headaches during the weekend and that "instead your subconscious mind will work out a dream which will help you understand your problem". On one occasion the patient graphically reported her sensa-

tions after such a suggestion as follows: "It seemed as though a dam had been erected in my mind to hold back a body of water. Every now and then there would be a gust of wind that splashed a little water over the dam and I would feel a twinge of pain, but then I would think to myself that I was not to have a headache and it would go away." There was never any evidence that the use of hypnosis in this way blocked the flow of material.

Discussion.

One of the noteworthy features of the case data is the almost exclusive preoccupation of the patient with so-called phallic material. It is probable that this is to a significant degree accounted for by the essentially hysterical nature of the illness. The personality development had apparently been basically sound, complicated only by the relatively circumscribed problems disclosed. But, to some extent, the relative absence in the patient's productions of material concerning problems other than phallic ones may be ascribed to the treatment method. Since the therapist was able to hold the patient to the problem at hand, digressions were relatively infrequent and this may have prevented the appearance of more material from other psychosexual levels, especially under the hypothesis that such material would arise as a resistance against the resolution of the regnant (phallic) conflict.

Another outstanding feature of the case data is the rapid translation of the patient's problems into their earlier childhood forms; the feeling of inferiority to men, for example, was first stated as inferiority in size, education, and opportunity but was soon translated into a feeling of inferiority because of the lack of a penis. Of course this regularly occurs in psychoanalysis but usually not so promptly. We would like to discuss several possible reasons for this quickened tempo, one more specific to this case and the other more generally applicable to hypnoanalysis.

The specific reason results from the fact that to this patient hypnosis meant the possibility of a realization of her fantasy of masochistic sexual surrender to a father-figure. Since this fantasy was an expression of one of her leading conflicts, the transference relationship almost at once duplicated the original neurosis, which then quickly appeared in its earlier form. It is also possible that the patient's wish for a penis, a hope frequently unconsciously entertained by women analysands, was here able to come more quickly to expression because of the magical power the patient ascribed to the hypnotist.

The reason generally regarded as chiefly responsible for the relative rapidity with which earlier and unconscious forms of the patient's conflict are revealed in hypnoanalysis is the circumventing of resistance in the hypnotic state. We would like to take up two frequently stated objections to hypnoanalysis which follow from this circumvention of resistance.

The first objection is that the failure to analyze the patient's problem in all of its current and conscious manifestations before plunging into its earlier and unconscious forms means that those manifestations not touched upon will remain unresolved and continue to give rise to symptoms. Against this objection is the fact that the patient reported in follow-up letters the disappearance of attitudes that had not been touched upon in the treatment. For example, she wrote that while nursing her son during an illness several months after her return home she suddenly realized that always in the past when she had mothered him she had felt strange and foreign, but that now this feeling of strangeness had disappeared. This feeling of strangeness was of course one manifestation of the patient's rejection of femininity, though it was never mentioned during treatment. It disappeared concomitantly with the general change in the patient's attitude toward her femininity.

The second objection is that hypnoanalysis can effect only very incomplete insight because it eliminates defenses instead of analyzing them. It is certainly not true that hypnosis eliminates defenses. It can weaken them and that only sometimes. More than one hour was spent in this case in a fruitless insistence that a particular dream symbol would be clarified or even that a particular dream would be recalled. The defense mechanism which seems to yield most readily to hypnosis is repression and it may be for this reason that hysteria—the neurosis in which repression is the dominant defense—is especially amenable to hypnoanalysis. Defense mechanisms can be analyzed in the hypnotic state just as in the waking state, and, with the material made available through the lifting of repression, perhaps more easily. How the hypnotic state affects defenses other than repression is an unexplored problem. If a patient in hypnosis can directly state the meaning of a dream, surely this means that the various defenses employed in the distortion of the latent dream-thought have somehow been altered.

With one incidental exception, the interviews with this patient were carried out entirely in the hypnotic state. This presents a very different picture of hypnotherapy from the sometimes described procedure in which material is obtained while the ego is held in abeyance and the material must subsequently be presented to the waking ego for any integration that takes place.

It is sometimes stated that the forcing of repressed material to consciousness would not be desirable even if it were possible because the unprepared ego would be unable to bear the anxiety provoked. The use of the technique of direct suggestion is a means of counteracting this anxiety. This patient responded very well to the suggestion that she would not consciously be concerned with her problems over the weekend, for example, and as already described her headaches were also sometimes handled in this way. We believe that the hypnotic relationship itself affords gratification and reassurance to the patient, since the therapist to some extent takes on himself the onus of responsibility for the material produced even though the patient must later accept the material as her own.

Another objection that has been raised against the forcing of repressed material into consciousness is that while this may lead to intellectual acceptance, emotional conviction is lacking.

In this case, however, the recovery of repressed material was accompanied by profound and appropriate affect, so that the hypnotic state appears to effect circumvention of the repression both of content and of affect. We have already discussed the use of regression to strengthen emotional insight.

A previous paper from this Clinic (4) has pointed out that a differentiation must be made between the changing transference manifestations as they take place during the course of the treatment and the relatively constant transference relationship which we assume to underlie the hypnotic state. That is, we assume that hypnotizability is essentially to be understood as a transference phenomenon and that a particular person can be hypnotized because the hypnotic relationship gratifies an unconscious fantasy or a wish, though this fantasy may vary from subject to subject. We had further assumed that in the course of hypnoanalytic therapy this fantasy could be explored and we would then know the basis of hypnotizability in this particular subject. We feel now, however, that a distinction must be made between the underlying basis of hypnotizability in a particular person and the meaning of hypnosis to that person. It is true that in a hypnoanalysis one can discover the meaning of hypnosis for a particular patient. It was clear in this patient that the hypnotic relationship meant a situation in which her masochistic fantasies might find expression, but it does not necessarily follow that this was why she was hypnotizable.

We feel that the distinction is of importance because it is of methodological significance in pursuing the question of the basis of hypnotizability. If hypnotizability were based on the gratification of a fantasy it might follow, for example, that the elucidation of this fantasy would lead to a change in the degree of hypnotizability. It has even been suggested that a "thoroughly" analyzed person would no longer be hypnotizable. It seems doubtful to us that even after a relatively prolonged and thorough analysis the basic unconscious fantasies are so altered that a previously existing hypnotizability would no longer be present. Certainly in this particular case the question cannot be decided if for no other reason than that the masochistic fantasies were only superficially explored.[2]

An undiscussed problem is the nature of the dreams which appear after direct suggestion in hypnosis, both those that take place that night during sleep and those that take place immediately in the hypnosis. Whether these dreams have any special characteristics and how they compare with ordinary dreams as well as the bearing of these hypnotically suggested dreams upon the problem of the relationship between hypnosis and sleep are unexplored problems.

Follow-up note: Two years after discharge this patient continued to be well and happy. In addition to carrying out her usual obligations she has achieved statewide and even some national recognition for her work in a women's organization.

[2] Although this topic cannot be pursued any further here, it should be pointed out that Kubie and Margolin have proposed a theory of hypnotizability which takes account of the transference phenomena existing in the hypnotic relationship without at the same time ascribing the hypnotizability to these transference phenomena. (5)

SELF-STARVATION AND COMPULSIVE HOPPING WITH PARADOXICAL REACTION TO HYPNOSIS [*]

BY MARGARET BRENMAN, PH.D.,

AND ROBERT P. KNIGHT, M.D.

When a psychiatric patient with an unusually bizarre symptom-picture that baffles understanding becomes an apparently hopeless therapeutic problem, and is then paradoxically started toward recovery by attempts at hypnosis which the patient requests to be terminated, one is impelled to give an account of such dramatic events. When, furthermore, subsequent psychotherapy provides material that illuminates the diagnosis, the psychodynamics, and the reasons for the previous therapeutic failures, one feels that much can be learned from reporting such a case in some detail. With these considerations in mind we present this report of a fourteen year old girl who is still in treatment but who has clinically recovered.

We shall relate first the present illness and clinical history as obtained upon admission, mainly from the mother; then give an account of the various treatment attempts which failed until the turning point came with attempted hypnosis; and, finally, present the illuminating material obtained from the patient herself during psychotherapy. A discussion of the diagnostic, psychodynamic, and child guidance aspects of the case concludes the paper.

Present Illness. The patient, an only child of fourteen, was brought to the Menninger Clinic by her parents mainly because they had reached an impasse in their efforts to feed her. She was 4 feet, 11 inches tall and weighed 70 pounds at the time of admission; she had lost 25 pounds in the three years

[*] Presented at the 1944 meeting, American Orthopsychiatric Association. Reprinted from *The American Journal of Orthopsychiatry,* Vol. XV, No. 1, January, 1945, pp. 65-75.

of her illness which began when she was eleven. Along with her refusal to eat, she had developed several bizarre compulsions. She would run everywhere instead of walk; at school she jumped up and down in her seat until she was severely bruised; she now refused to sit down in most situations; and finally, she had begun to hop violently on her right leg for hours at a time. At fourteen she was still not menstruating nor had she developed any secondary sexual characteristics.

Historical sketch. Most of the historical background was obtained from the mother, an artificially gay and talkative woman. Admitting it was not her nature to be affectionate, she said she had rarely kissed her little girl, even as a baby. She described the patient as always having conformed to her own mother's ideal of a girl: "Neat, a lady, and good at the piano." She added that the child had always had an excellent appetite and was an example in this regard for other children in the neighborhood. She was a model child, never broke a toy and was always obedient. Her only problem had been lifelong constipation. Like her father, she was meticulous about her personal belongings and was a great collector of coins, pocketbooks, stamps, charms, dogs, and the like. Quite incidentally the mother mentioned that the patient's first three years at school had been hampered by frequent attacks of asthma and that for a short time she had been placed on a restricted diet. The importance to the patient of this enforced dieting was not seen until it was discussed by the patient herself during the later psychotherapy. In spite of these interruptions, she had maintained an "A" average in school until the present illness began at eleven. As the asthmatic attacks subsided in her twelfth year, the feeding difficulties of the present illness began.

The father's business kept him away from home several days each week. Being an only child, the patient was thrown into close contact with her mother. The father was very fond of the patient who, in turn, according to the mother, "worshipped" him. He had been inclined to make light of the patient's illness, saying that she would outgrow these silly habits.

Patient was first observed striking her head against the pillow when she was eleven years old, shortly after the mother was taken to the hospital for abdominal surgery. During her mother's sixteen weeks' absence the patient did not see her but asked no questions and seemed relatively unconcerned. However, she began to have restless and apparently troubled nights and could not fall asleep until she had pounded her head backwards on the pillow many times. After the mother's return from the hospital, the patient began refusing to eat. At first her mother would only guide the spoon to the patient's mouth, but soon she was spoon-feeding her entirely. At the age of twelve she began to hop with increasing violence and frequency.

For three years the mother waged a losing battle. Patient became increasingly resistive to being fed; she clawed, kicked, and spat the food from her mouth. Except for several brief periods of improvement her hopping became more frantic and continuous. She was taken to a clinic in a midwestern metropolis where a clitoral circumcision was performed "in order to decrease her nervousness". When it became obvious that this had no such effect, she was taken to the Mayo Clinic where it was recommended, in the absence of any positive physical findings, that she be referred to the Menninger Clinic for psychiatric study and treatment.

During the psychological examination, the patient gave terse factual answers to direct questions and maintained an emotionally flat reserve throughout. No fantasies or dreams could be elicited. Psychological tests showed her to be of distinctly superior intelligence with, however, serious impairment of concentration. This latter finding was reflected in the fact that her grades had dropped from an A average to C's and D's.

When the case was discussed by the staff, the diagnosis of severe compulsion neurosis prevailed slightly over schizophrenia and the prognosis was considered to be extremely guarded.

Treatment Attempts.

1.   Southard School (one week); attempted psychoanalysis with woman analyst (four months). Patient was first admitted to the children's service of the Clinic of the Southard School, and daily interviews with a woman child-analyst were arranged. Throughout her stay at the School she was abnormally docile, polite in an artificial and stilted way, and almost totally devoid of appropriate emotional reaction. She talked guardedly and sparingly with the analyst. She flatly refused nourishment or hid her food in the yard. Hopping became even more violent, and her weight continued to drop alarmingly. Life saving measures became necessary and she was transferred to the Sanitarium for tube-feeding and general hospital care.

2.   Sanitarium care; male analyst (one month). Compulsive hopping now grew so violent that she was constantly drenched in perspiration and seemed on the verge of total exhaustion. To avert this she was placed in a cold pack for certain daily periods. Although at first she accepted the tube-feeding with little protest, she became increasingly resistant to any type of hospital care and frequently kicked over the tube-feeding. She began to gain weight from the feedings and complained of this bitterly. With her increased combativeness, it soon took three nurses to put her into the pack, and during these struggles this 90 pound girl injured several of them and even bruised two male attendants. She abandoned all interest in her general bodily care and fiercely fought attempts to bathe her or to deal with her unkempt appearance. Because she had remained inaccessible during her analytic hours with a "mother-figure" analyst, she was transferred to a male analyst. After a month of patient effort he, too, found her inaccessible. She had taken what appeared to be a psychotic attitude toward her symptoms, stoutly maintaining that she was not sick and that her behavior was in no way unusual. By this time she presented a more severe problem in institutional management than any other patient in the Sanitarium. Since the general feeling was that the prognosis was growing more grave, it was

decided that should she fail to respond to a final plan of treatment, it would be recommended to her parents that she be removed to a state hospital for custodial care.

3.   Sanitarium care; turning point with attempted hypnosis (two days). This final plan included trial interviews in hypnosis by one of the authors (M. B.) with supervision by the other (R. P. K.). At first she was as resistive to this as to all previous approaches, but finally agreed to cooperate if she were permitted to hop for a certain period each day. This "bargain" made, the patient went into a light hypnosis for an hour on each of two successive days while in the pack. During these hours an extremely permissive attitude was adopted by the therapist who suggested simply that her general tension and restlessness would decrease so that she would not need to hop so violently. When taken out of the pack after the second interview preparatory to going for her hopping session, she attempted to jump and suddenly cried, "I can't jump any more!" She continued to try and succeeded in jumping violently for a short time during her scheduled "jumping time". When she returned to the Sanitarium she screamed, "They have done something to me! I can't jump any more! It's terrible, it's terrible, what shall I do!" She ran about wildly, screaming, and suddenly threw pillows and bedding across the room, smashed toilet articles and stamped on them, and even tried to toss the mattress off the bed but found her strength unequal to it. This tempestuous outburst marked the turning point in her treatment. It ended the hopping symptom but she continued to refuse to eat, to dress and undress, to bathe, and to sit or lie down until she was put to bed by the nurse.

4.   Sanitarium care; companion therapy (four-and-a-half weeks). The following day she met the therapist's attempt to hypnotize her with the statement that there was surely no further need to carry out this procedure inasmuch as she was no longer hopping. When asked whether she did not believe the fact that she was being tube-fed was still something of a problem, she became coldly polite and evasive. Further tactful

attempts to convince her she should go on with hypnosis were met with statements like "I don't believe so", or "Perhaps it's not really necessary". It appeared that she regarded hypnosis as a powerful threat to her remaining symptoms and that she was not yet ready to abandon the tube-feeding. The therapist did not press the issue and suggested instead that she would continue to come to visit the patient anyway. Although by no means enthusiastic about this latter plan, patient did not oppose it, but said: "But, you know, I really don't need any analysis. I've gone all through that twice now."

During the following four and a half weeks no concerted attack on her refusal to eat was made. She was taken for walks outside the Sanitarium grounds. On rainy days she was taught chess. She agreed to sit down for the chess games with the therapist, and felt this to be a distinct concession, inasmuch as it was her determined policy to stand up until she literally dropped with exhaustion into a chair, and had to be undressed and put to bed. Occasionally the therapist introduced the general topic of food in an oblique way, and gradually the patient became willing to discuss menus in the abstract. Also she was frequently observed reading food advertisements and articles on meal-planning in magazines.

5. Sanitarium care; psychotherapy. During this period the patient attempted many kinds of strategy. At first she took the position that she was cured and very eager to go home to her parents, giving ingenious arguments to support her declared belief that it would be quite all right to be spoon-fed by her mother for the rest of her life. Then she attempted to play her hospital physician (also a woman) and the therapist against each other, telling the former that she felt her psychotherapy sessions were a waste of time because "we never talk about the eating" and yet refusing with great irritation to discuss the problem with the therapist whenever it was broached. She begged her hospital physician for electro-shock treatments, saying that if she were granted these she would probably start to eat because it would prove that we regarded her as an im-

portant adult. She felt that "these talking treatments are only for kids" and that "the other ladies on the floor aren't treated by just talking unless they have a very small problem". When this proposal was rejected she began to suggest experimental bargains, such as letting her go for two or three weeks without any feedings at all; this, she felt, would surely make her hungry enough to want to eat. Accordingly, on two occasions she was allowed to go for forty-eight hours without a tube-feeding. This, however, brought no significant result.

In spite of these elaborate attempts to mislead and outwit her hospital physician and therapist, she was becoming increasingly communicative. She began to participate tentatively in the exploration of the feelings she had had when her illness began. The day before she determined to start eating again, we had discussed, on an extremely generalized level, the fact that sometimes one may have feelings for one's mother other than pure love. Although she became extremely tense during this hour, she concluded by saying that sometimes she felt she might start to eat again, but not yet. The therapist pointed out that the hospital physician, of whom the patient was very fond, was becoming tired of the tube-feedings, and that several staff members had suggested that the patient be returned to the children's division. The mere mention of this possibility frightened her, and at first she became enraged at the therapist for telling her. Then she began to cry and plead with the therapist for help. This was the first genuine display of appropriate emotion she had made. She burst into a tirade against "the kind of psychiatry they use down at the School", saying: "The whole week I was there they just let me go without trying to get me to eat . . . nobody cared, just indifferent. It was real mental torture." It became quite clear from this hour and from material elicited much later in treatment that the patient's need for absolute infantile dependence was intense, and that the laissez-faire attitude which had deliberately been adopted at the School, had produced an agony of insecurity. She now decided to start eating in order to avert a repetition of being thus thrown on her own resources. At the Sanitarium she could maintain the illusion of being an adult, whereas at the School she felt she would be regarded as "one of the kids", but feared actually that she would be less directly protected and cared for. She was handled skillfully by her hospital physician who allayed her still present fear of eating by agreeing to put her on a "reducing diet". She was greatly pleased by this, for she had gained 25 pounds as a result of the tube-feedings. It is curious that along with her decision to eat she determined to learn to smoke.

A period of literal gluttony now followed during which the patient's demands for food were insatiable. She talked of almost nothing but the wonderful experience of eating and invented fantastic dishes for herself, such as a bag of peanuts poured into a malted milk and flavored with grape soda pop. Although these extravagant splurges alarmed her occasionally, she was reassured. She continued to eat whatever she was impelled to, although she felt she could never be really satisfied.[1] At the same time, she began to take a real interest in her appearance—she experimented with new coiffures, began to use cosmetics and to manicure her nails.

For several weeks after she had begun to eat, she took the stand that now she was really cured and was eager to go home to her parents. However, she continued to refuse to open their letters or to write to them. Very haltingly she began to confess vague feelings of hostility, particularly toward her mother, finally admitting that she preferred not to go home "ever". She fantasied going to live "in a boarding house where I won't get attached to anyone".

The history of her dieting, mentioned casually by her mother as an inconsequential period when she was a youngster, was given quite a different emphasis by the patient. She felt that her present eating splurges were an attempt to "make up" for a lifetime of deprivation. She described with both humor and bitterness the endless series of diets with which her mother

---

[1] At no time did the patient show any allergic reactions to food of any type during the many months she was under treatment.

had attempted to meet the presumed allergic condition. First there would be a period of nothing but fruits; then no fruit, and nothing but vegetables; and at one time, "I was left with nothing but seven-minute cabbage." Many strange and non-sensical variations of protein and carbohydrate balances, concocted by so-called "Health Institutes" were tried for a time. Certain constants were maintained in all of these restricted menus: eggs, milk or anything presumed to have milk in it (ice-cream, candy, and so forth), had been forbidden for as long as she could remember. Cake was taboo as well, because wheat flour was regarded by the mother as poisonous for the patient. She sometimes let herself eat these snacks at parties "just to be devilish". Thus oral pleasure became bound up with wickedness, rebellion, and guilt.

The patient's revelations regarding her diet history seemed at such odds with the mother's casual statement that further inquiry was made of the mother. Although this information was difficult to elicit, it soon appeared that the patient's version was substantially accurate. The mother described her conscientious efforts to find the right doctor to treat the patient's asthma; she recalled that when the patient was eight she had gone to a well-known physician who had recommended no diet regulation. She added: "I couldn't work with him at all." She attributed to "mother's intuition" her decision to place milk, eggs, and wheat in the tabooed category, and she spoke with nostalgia of "the days when my little girl was so nice and fat and rosy".

The patient herself regarded the time when she was fat with no such nostalgia, and recalled with aversion being teased and called "Fatty" by her schoolmates. The problem of weight gain had grown out of all proportion for her. Clearly, this problem is rooted in conflicts far deeper than either the mother's oral preoccupation or the fact of schoolmates' teasing. But the patient did not approach a discussion of these conflicts until some time after she had been discharged from the Sanitarium and placed in a foster home. This change in her status was not attempted until six months after she had first begun to eat.

6. Foster home placement; return to public school (continued psychotherapy). Although she was attached to the Sanitarium and reluctant to leave, she has made a good adjustment to her foster home and to public school. Her grades are high and she is sought out by her schoolmates. She still prefers the company of adults, and rationalizes this by the adoption of superior and scornful attitudes toward "the kids". Her eating habits are somewhat erratic since she has been controlling them herself, and she has by no means yet worked through this problem. She still makes a careful distinction between "regular meals" and "snacks", and is constantly driven in the direction of eating between meals, although not without guilt. She has maintained her body weight and is in good health.

Since her placement in a foster home, she has been seen regularly in psychotherapeutic interviews, and is making an earnest attempt to go back through the history of her illness "to prevent its ever happening again". She is increasingly spontaneous in the discussions and often returns to painful memories because "it's better to talk it out". By far the most striking of these were her recollections of the onset of her illness. She felt that she had "begun to get funny ideas" long before her mother went to the hospital. Secretly she would go to her room and stand before a picture of her father with his arm around her; she would think how intensely she loved him, meanwhile smiling at the picture and patting a jewel-box he had given her. It was during this ritual that she had first begun to hop. She had felt herself becoming increasing religious; she could not go to sleep until she had recited a prayer in which she begged God to take care of her parents and to give her a good day, emphasizing the prayer by beating her head on the pillow. She climaxed these confessions by saying that finally she had come to the conclusion that she was really the "daughter of God", and as such she must lead a pure life of sacrifice and distasteful exertion, to achieve and maintain the supernatural power which would be proper to a daughter of God. Hopping was the "extra work" which a member of the holy family would be expected to do. She had decided that in this chosen capacity she must surely be different from other girls and would thus never menstruate. She explicitly related this belief to her intense feelings for her father and felt it was a way of maintaining the status quo.

In discussing this delusion the patient repeatedly used scornful and mocking phrases and felt she had never had any real attachment to her parents, inasmuch as her present feeling was one of pure hate. She added that when she was brought to the Sanitarium this "foolish idea" was still firmly entrenched. She was in constant dread that the analysts, whom she regarded as having a supernatural power similar to her own, might ferret out her secret. She had given up this idea only gradually as her feelings for her father had subsided. She felt that as the daughter of God she would probably be seated at his left, "because Jesus was already on his right", and added that in some ill-defined way this would be "crowding Mother out". It was in this setting that her mother became ill.

At first, the patient was delighted with the fact that temporarily the roles were reversed. She took care of her mother while she was still at home, and even fed her. But when her mother became gravely ill and was taken to the hospital, the patient suffered acute guilt because she felt it was her fault. In recalling these feelings she suddenly remembered that she had been playing with a kitten just before her mother was taken away, and had not put it back with its mother but had left it by the roadside. She felt that symbolically she had separated a mother and child, and was punished for this by being separated from her own mother.

In spite of the burden of the belief that it was she who was responsible for her mother's absence, patient says there was much satisfaction in that period "because I had Dad all to myself". It was not until her mother returned home that her refusal to eat began. She felt that this and her head-banging were attempts to fight back. Although her hopping had originated as part of the ritual in front of her father's picture, she now believes that gradually she had decided to use it as an auxiliary weapon to her refusal to eat, as a method of "staying real thin".

It has become increasingly clear that one of the nuclear factors in this desperate effort to prevent weight gain was the struggle against growing up. The patient states that she wanted things to remain "just the way they were", above all in her relationship to her father. Being slim meant to her simply not getting any "bigger". She now recognized her reluctance to grow up, and pointed out that it must be an important problem to her, since at fifteen she is not yet menstruating. She feels that "sex is a great mystery—and sort of scary", in spite of the fact that her actual information on this subject is somewhat more complete than that possessed by the average adolescent. Her earlier nightmares of terrified flight from masked bandits have given way to dreams in which, for example, she sees herself at a dance with a boy from school. She is struck by the fact that in her dream she chooses "one of the poor, rough, dirty boys instead of a nice one", and quickly adds: "That must mean I sort of still think of sex as dirty and bad, deep down." This frank coming to grips with her problems is in sharpest contrast to the earlier complete denial of her most obvious symptoms. It is hoped that further development of insight will fortify her against a repetition of her illness when she attempts later to make an adult heterosexual adjustment.

Discussion.

The discussion of this case will include a consideration of several interrelated but distinct problems. 1) The question of diagnosis; 2) the psychodynamics thus far revealed; 3) the problem of the patient's reactions to treatment attempts and especially the paradoxical reaction to hypnosis; 4) the special role played by the overemphasis on diet in this and similar cases.

Although the diagnosis of "severe compulsion neurosis" prevailed slightly over schizophrenia when the patient was first
discussed by the staff, her subsequent behavior, as well as the
content of the material elicited in the psychotherapy, makes
this differential diagnosis even more difficult. Her performance
on the psychological tests[2] was characteristically compulsive.
She gave pedantically sharp and deliberate responses and,
although there was marked impairment of concentration, there
was no sign of schizophrenic disorganization in any of the tests.
These findings, together with the clinical picture at the time of
admission, militate against a diagnosis of schizophrenia. An
additional line of evidence which brings this case closer to
the compulsion neuroses is its resemblance to the syndrome
"anorexia nervosa" recently described as occurring in an obsessive or compulsive personality more frequently than in any
other group (14) (15).

When the presenting symptoms are limited to this syndrome,
anorexia nervosa has lately been regarded as a separate disease
entity. When it has been found together with other symptoms
it has been thought of as simply a symptomatic diagnosis. The
status of this diagnostic category reflects the present nosological confusion between purely descriptive and dynamically
conceived psychiatric categories. There is, however, fairly
unanimous agreement that the three primary symptoms found
to be pathognomonic for anorexia nervosa as a clinical description are the rejection of food, constipation, and amenorrhea.
All three were present in our patient. Moreover, the psychological background of recently studied cases of anorexia
nervosa, and the dramatization of the underlying conflicts
through the specific symptoms enumerated, are clearly paralleled in this case. The importance of noting this similarity is
not that it provides yet another possible diagnostic label, but
rather that it might serve to clarify further the status of the

2 The following nine psychological tests were administered: Stanford-Binet,
Form L; Cornell-Coxe Performance Test; Wechsler-Bellevue Scale; Rorschach;
Szondi; Hanfmann-Kasanin, and B.R.L. Concept Formation tests; Thematic
Apperception, and Association Tests.

term anorexia nervosa as a descriptive rather than a dynamically conceived category. It is difficult to place this case, even
on a descriptive level, with the anorexia nervosas because of
the severity of the patient's regression, together with the discovery of a clear-cut delusion. Thus, the problem of final diagnosis remains an open question.

As in the recently reported anorexia nervosas, the essential
economic aim of this patient's illness has been to block normal
"growing up", with its attendant threat of being forced to
abandon intense oedipal fantasies and to accept genital sexuality. Our patient states this proposition in the following way:
"When I came to the Clinic I couldn't talk to the analyst about
being the daughter of God because I thought they'd try to
talk me out of it; and that would mean giving up all those
feelings about my father, and I knew I didn't want to." In
this setting of an intense oedipal conflict, the patient's mother
was eliminated from the scene by illness. Patient attempted
to deal with her severe guilt feelings while her mother was in
the hospital by the series of compulsive undoing mechanisms
and rituals described earlier—banging her head while praying,
hopping, and so forth. Her refusal to eat began only after her
mother had returned; she herself regards this as an expression
of her rage and defiance against her mother for again interfering with her relationship to her father. She says that she adopted this avenue of attack because "eating was always so important to Mother and she had always bragged on me for
being such a good eater". At the same time, she was enabled
to escape her great anxiety by regressing to a level of extreme
infantile dependence in being spoon-fed, and still express her
resentment against her mother by her uncooperativeness in
being fed. There has been as yet no evidence for believing
that this anxiety was further aggravated by fantasies of oral
impregnation. We mention this because in the cases referred
to such fantasies have been regularly observed.

We come now to a summary of the therapeutic approaches
made, and to the discussion of the possible reasons for the

failure of the earlier, and the success of the later, attempts. When the patient was first admitted to the Southard School, the decision to adopt a laissez-faire policy in regard to her eating was made on the assumption that a further extension of the pitched battle between the patient and her mother would be useless. It now appears that this treatment resulted only in a sense of panic and insecurity in this child, giving her the feeling that she was left completely vulnerable to the onslaughts of her own instinctual demands. Her desperate defense was an uncompromising self-starvation. When the threat to her life became evident, it was necessary to adopt an opposite attitude in her management. She was forced to eat by tube-feeding, and at the same time was blocked in her symptom outlet of hopping, in order to prevent further exhaustion and weight loss. Although no doubt she was profoundly relieved that adults had once more "taken over the controls" she felt at the same time a surge of rage and defiance at being completely deprived of her earlier defenses—and at being forced to gain weight and thus "grow up". It was impossible, and to an extent still is difficult for her to tolerate any but an illusional kind of growing up. In this framework the analysts were simply representatives of the enemy inasmuch as they sometimes talked to her about her future. She felt they were intent on making her give up her father, thus she could have no communication with them. She felt, too, that they constantly gave her the impression that any changes which would take place would be entirely her own responsibility. This was a terrifying prospect.

The trial interviews in hypnosis came at a propitious time. Her anxiety at having gained 25 pounds was becoming intolerable; she said: "I was so sick of fighting but I couldn't give in." She regarded hypnosis as "something magical" and felt that it would force her to a change. Although this prospect was frightening, it shifted the responsibility from her to an omnipotent adult. Her dramatic response to the implied suggestion that she would give up hopping reinforced her belief that hypnosis was indeed a powerful threat to her symptoms, and

she declined to cooperate any further. But the necessary leverage to her recovery had already been achieved. Eissler (9) has
described a strikingly similar experience in the treatment of a
case of anorexia nervosa in which contact was established by a
magical device after many "rational" approaches had failed.
It is as if a deep regression must sometimes be met with an
attack which appears to the patient adequate to it. This is the
primitive and archaic language of magic. Once the critical
shift away from the psychotic inaccessibility had been established, it seemed not only unnecessary but impolitic to continue with this technique when the patient regarded it as such
a powerful threat.

Accordingly, her anxiety was allayed by temporarily giving
up the attack on her symptoms and by sustaining her in an
atmosphere of strong but permissive protection. The nurses
were instructed to be particularly friendly and affectionate
at this time. When the patient was then faced with the possibility of being returned to the Southard School, she envisioned
it as a threat to her new-found security and determined to start
eating.

With gradual maneuvering back into life via a foster home,
there came the opening up of conflict material which is en-
abling the patient to see with increasing clarity the ambiguity
of her adjustment. She now admits that although she plays
at being an adult in her smoking and her requests for "rum-
cokes" and beer, she is actually frightened of the main business
of growing up insofar as it involves such experiences as menstruating, having dates, and ultimately marrying.

In conclusion, we should like to suggest some of the practical implications which may be drawn from the study of this
and similar cases mentioned. It is evident that the mother's
preoccupation with food and diet control has in every instance
contributed significantly to the precipitation of the severe eating disorder. It is as though the establishment by the mother
of many taboo areas of oral gratification is seen by the child
as equivalent to a deprivation of love, and thus re-awakens

infantile oral conflicts. Simultaneously, it provides the child with a weapon of unparalleled strength when there arises a conflict with the mother, a weapon that then threatens the child's own survival. Quite specifically, it would appear that in many cases of so-called allergic reactions (asthma, in our patient) psychotherapy with the mother would be indicated rather than an attempt at rigid diet control in the child. The physician and the parents must find and maintain that delicate balance of indulgence and restraint that exactly fits the particular emotional needs and anxieties of the individual child. This is usually arrived at by the "good parent" through a process of trial-and-error. The study of cases such as this brings us closer to an understanding of how such a balance may be struck and what kinds of advice we should give parents.

If we can, through case studies of this kind, sharpen the alertness of both physicians and parents to the emotional factors in eating disorders, it will be possible to institute proper psychotherapeutic management before the child is driven into psychotic regression by the intensity of the oral conflicts. Perhaps it is only through such an educational campaign that we will be able to reverse the present dismal prognosis generally given to severe anorexias.[3]

Follow-up note: Psychotherapy was continued with progressively decreasing frequency for another year, during the last of which she was seen on an average of once every three weeks. During the past year, she has been seen once at her request following a stressful "break" with a girl-friend. Her relation to her parents has become normally warm and friendly and she leads an active extra-curricular life. Her mother has written us that menses have begun and that the patient has shown no unusual reactions. Except for some continued food fads and shyness with boys, her general adjustment is very good. It is now three years since she was discharged from the hospital.

[3] Acknowledgment is due Dr. E. M. Leitch of the staff of the Menninger Clinic for her cooperation in the study of this case.

AN EXPERIMENTAL STUDY

The Use of Hypnotic Techniques in a Study of Tension Systems[*]

BY MARGARET BRENMAN, PH.D.

I. *Introduction: Statement of the Problem*

The broadest aim of this research is to contribute to the attempt to cope with the recognized dilemma of "vitality of material versus precision of method" by illustrating the use of hypnosis as a tool of experiment in conjunction with a relatively standardized technique developed by experimental psychology. Before detailing the nature of the specific problem, several theoretical considerations are in order, inasmuch as this presentation is an attempt to clarify certain theoretical problems as well as to report tentative experimental findings.

It is easier and perhaps less ambiguous to construct an experiment within the "theory" of a single school of psychology where the aims have already been clearly established, where an accepted terminology has been invented, and where specific procedures have been devised to the end of studying certain kinds of problems. Yet it has been precisely this internal systematization within each school which has contributed to the stalemate of the science of psychology. The volume of critical discussions of methodology and of the applications of the philosophy of science to the particular discipline of psychology clearly shows the increasing awareness that the isolated monopolies in psychological research must give way to an integration of the most fruitful theories, tools, and experimental procedures. Such an integration must not be simply a superficial eclecticism in which an experimenter blindly picks from a scientific grab-bag whatever theories or procedures

* This study is a condensed version of a thesis submitted to the Department of Psychology and the Faculty of the Graduate School of the University of Kansas in May, 1942, in partial fulfillment of the requirements for the degree of Doctor of Philosophy.

seemed most convenient for his problem of the moment. Rather, there must be evolved a highly systematized theoretical framework which can dictate the construction of a specific experiment. In such a system, such constructs as "drive", "tension system" and "instinctual striving" would be unequivocally differentiated from each other, united in a single clear-cut concept, or abandoned. It is obvious that such an advance in methodological sophistication will not result simply from a preoccupation with the verbal-logical problems of extending a speculative blue-print system nor from an emphasis on what Pratt (37) has aptly called the "formal" properties of an observed event. A slow and painstaking series of experiments, specifically designed to meet the present urgent need for systematic integration, will be prerequisite to this growth. This is not to say that the development of theory must wait for the lagging experiment; it is simply a restatement of the well-known fact that, "theory without practice is sterile, practice without theory is blind."

The present investigation has been conceived against the background of its historical position in the development of the science of psychology as an example of the kind of study which may contribute to the closing of "schisms" within the science of psychology. J. F. Brown (8) (9) (10) has discussed in detail the fundamental trends in the history of psychology since the days when both psychology, under Wundt's leadership, and psychiatry, led by Kraepelin, were agreed that atomistic classification was all-important. He has shown that, from the time of the split which followed Freud's early work up to the present, there has been a consistent contrast between the rich content but methodological weakness in the psychoanalytic approach on the one hand, and the increasing methodological precision but weakness in "vital interest" of general experimental psychology on the other. He has shown further that the conceptual development of Gestalt psychology in general, and of Lewinian psychology in particular, has been paralleled by the independent and fertile development of psychoanalysis; and that the current trend in experimental psychopathology is toward a resolution of the breach between these two. Lewin (28) has also discussed the points of similarity in these two approaches; although this comparison and contrast will be further developed later on, it should be stated at the outset that both theoretical approaches accept the modern organismic position, whether by implication as in psychoanalytic theory or by frequent concrete statement as in Gestalt and Lewinian theory. It is this fundamental philosophical agreement that has made possible cooperative research problems between the two and without which the present transitional period could not have come about.

The essentially transitional character of the present study will be readily seen in the variety of sources upon which it has had to draw, first in order to establish some "frame of reference" for the problem and secondly for specific techniques of experiment. We have found it necessary to survey again the problem of "memory", the traditional property of the experimental psychologist, only recently pried loose from the "associationist". Modifications of the "Zeigarnik technique",[1] one of the most famous investigations of motivation in memory, were adopted as the nucleus of our procedures. Hypnosis, a tool developed mainly by the clinician, was the vehicle of the investigation. Finally, the nucleus of the problem, namely the attempt to derive from these procedures some hint regarding influence of the motivational factors on recall and on preferred activity, has for the most part been considered most fruitfully probed by the psychoanalysts. The specific application to the present problem of these various "ways and means" will be elaborated later on; they have been mentioned in order to illustrate the extreme catholicity of selection which was necessary

[1] B. Zeigarnik, a student of Kurt Lewin, gave subjects a number of tasks to do but permitted them to complete only half of these. She then asked the subjects to recall as many of the tasks as they could and found that the interrupted tasks had a significant memory advantage. She concluded from this that a "tension system" had been set up and that the intention or need to complete the interrupted tasks was evidenced in the fact that they were better remembered (51). This study will be discussed in detail later on.

to carry forward the investigation of a problem which might explore an area common to psychoanalytic and Lewinian theory.

This selection of ways and means was determined further by a consideration of the problem of "vitality versus precision" of experiment. Lewin (29) has made it clear that this situation is not necessarily a dilemma without a solution. He has expressed his hope for psychology in the following:

> " . . . The psychologist finds himself in the midst of a rich and vast land full of strange happenings: there are men killing themselves; a child playing; a child forming his lips trying to say his first word; a person who having fallen in love and being caught in an unhappy situation is not willing or not able to find a way out; there is the mystical state called hypnosis, where the will of one person seems to govern another person; there is the reaching out for higher, and more difficult goals; loyalty to a group; dreaming; planning; exploring the world; and so on without end. It is an immense continent full of fascination and power and full of stretches of land where no one has ever set foot.
>
> "Psychology is out to conquer this continent, to find out where its treasures are hidden, to investigate its danger spots, to master its vast forces, and to utilize its energies."

Thus Lewin expresses his belief that it is not impossible to ultimately develop methods whereby vital phenomena may be attacked by precise experiments.

We have stated that the present exploratory study is an attempt to illustrate one kind of experiment aimed at bridging the gap between clinical observation and experiment, and between general psychology and psychoanalytic theory. It is no more than that. Glib "proofs" or "disproofs" of psychoanalytic theory simply do lip-service to this end; this theory cannot be proven or disproven by a single experiment nor by a dozen experiments. The many attempts to produce such simple "proofs" or "disproofs" as we shall see have usually done little more than reveal a general naiveté of general psychology with regard to psychoanalytic theory. A substantial and valid rapprochement between the two disciplines will be accomplished only by a long-term systematic exploration of phenomena related to those observed phenomena upon which psychoanalytic theory has been built. The investigations reported here are but tentative moves in that direction.

II. *Background of the Problem*

We have surveyed four types of investigation to provide the background for the present study: (1) theoretical discussions of the relation of psychology and psychoanalysis; (2) studies usually described as inquiries into the "influence of emotions on memory"; (3) investigations that have employed hypnosis as a research tool; and (4) studies by Lewin and his pupils related specifically to the problem of motivational factors in memory and task-resumption, and more generally to the problem of integrating psychoanalytic theory with Lewinian psychology.

(1) Critical Discussions of Psychology and Psychoanalysis

Although on the whole it has been the academic psychologist and not the psychoanalyst who has been concerned with the problems of "conceptual refinement" and general methodology, the recognition of common problems and of the need for systematization in psychology has not been entirely confined to the academician. Yet, despite several noteworthy attempts at conciliation from each "camp", the present situation still precludes a genuine and consistent working relationship between them.

Brown (8) (9) (10) and Lewin (28) have discussed at length the important similarities and differences between the topological and the psychoanalytic approaches. These were only indicated in the introduction. Both agree that in each approach there is implicit an organismic philosophy which necessitates the breakdown of dichotomies, a central interest in the underlying significance of *all* psychological phenomena, and a belief that the development of a multiple-structured personality results from a process of differentiation and integration of parts out of primitive wholes. Both agree, too, that there are serious differences between the two approaches which might be resolved by cooperative research. The essential differences emphasized are these: first psychoanalytic theory has been built on the basis of clinical observation while that of topological psychology has been built on precisely constructed experiments; secondly, psychoanalysis has neglected logical strictness of theory (a nuclear factor in topological psychology) and is thus, according to Lewin (28), "a *body of ideas* rather than a *system of theories* and concepts"; and finally, psychoanalysis does not sharply distinguish between historical and systematic problems and tends to favor the former type of description. This last point has been emphasized by Lewin who has suggested that here perhaps lies the crux of the problem.

One might suppose that the psychoanalyst would judge this last mentioned problem of little practical importance, and find it difficult to accept even as a theoretical proposition. Yet the question of "historical" versus "ahistorical" emphases has recently been the topic of heated debate between various groups of psychoanalysts. It has come to expression in Horney's (22) contrast of "horizontal" with "vertical" analysis. Alexander (3) in a critical discussion of the need for the revision of psychoanalytic theory has suggested that:

"Horney's error lies in erecting an antithesis between the analysis of the actual dynamic structure of the patient . . . as opposed to the genetic point of view . . . only both points of view together can give a satisfactory understanding of human behavior."[2]

Alexander states further that:

"Freud was primarily a great observer and only secondarily a great theoretician. His theories sometimes lack strict consistency, contain contradictions, and are avowedly of a preliminary nature. One must realize that he did pioneer work in an almost virgin territory. He developed an extremely refined instrument for psychological investigations, accumulated novel observations, and it is only natural that his first formulations were groping attempts to bring some order into the chaos of the newly discovered field of

[2] p. 18.

the dynamics of human personality. He was perfectly aware of the shortcomings of his theoretical concepts and . . . consistently worked on their improvement. He justifiably stated that it was too early to create a pedantic and strictly defined conceptual system because this would hamper further development."[3]

This quotation is evidence against the current belief that psychoanalysts have no awareness of the methodological crisis existing in the science of psychology and that they adhere in a slavish and satisfied fashion to the concepts originally set up by Freud.

Further evidence for a growing sensitivity among psychoanalysts to the need for "improving the method" is provided in a suggestive discussion by Bernfeld (6). He argues that scientific methods are always specializations and refinements of everyday common-sense techniques; and applying this fact to psychoanalysis, he concludes that everyday conversation has provided the basic model for psychoanalytic techniques. It is his opinion that conversation is a model hitherto used but little in science and therefore subject to great scorn and skepticism by non-analytically oriented scientists. He proposes, then, systematic experimental studies of the "psychology or the logic of conversation" which would investigate specifically the conditions under which obstacles to communication may be removed and the relation of such findings to the "solution of resistance" in psychoanalysis. He says:

"Theoretically, such experiments are not impossible, though practically they will be difficult—and fascinating. The recent development of experimental psychology has shown that ingenuity has overcome obstacles to experimentation which formerly appeared to be unsurmountable. The work of Lewin and his pupils, which in many respects is related to the program we are speaking of, is an example."[4]

[3] pp. 25-26.

[4] p. 305.

Bernfeld, commenting on the necessity for developing new techniques in experimental psychology to meet the problems raised by psychoanalytic theory, says wittily: "What we see through the microscope we cannot check by eye-glasses." He develops this further, saying:

"The observations made by the technique cannot and need not be checked by other, so-called usual, methods. Insofar as psychoanalysis uses techniques equivalent to new observation instruments, it is not subject to the approved 'other methods.' "[5]

This statement, although intended by its author as a warning comment with regard to future experimentation, is a succinct and appropriate criticism of the body of experiments designed by general psychologists to prove or disprove Freudian theory. This will be seen in greater detail in the section devoted to "Experimental Studies".

It has been mentioned that the points of contact between psychoanalytic theory and general psychology occur at the intersection provided by the organismic philosophy or generalized "field-theory". An excellent illustration of the extent to which the conceptual approach and even the terminology of field-theory have been accepted by some workers in psychoanalysis is a paper by Thomas M. French, entitled, "Goal, Mechanism, and Integrative Field" (20) in which he begins:

"The aim of psychoanalysis is the study of human motives. A motive is a concept that implies striving toward a goal. Everyone knows that rational behavior has a purposive goal-seeking character. Psychoanalysis has demonstrated that irrational behavior also is striving, though less successfully, toward the fulfillment of wishes."[6]

He elaborates this view in a well-documented, scholarly discussion, giving a "dynamic analysis of goal-directed behavior".

[5] p. 303.
[6] p. 226.

The following quotation, taken from the body of this paper, represents the quality of the entire argument and is given here because it shows so unambiguously the impact on psychoanalytic thought of recent advances in the theoretical systems developed by general psychology, specifically by the "field-theorists":

> "As we have seen, the goal-directed striving acting through the medium of a cognitive field, must successively activate one subsidiary goal after another and inhibit other goal-directed strivings, all in accordance with the time-schedule contained in the cognitive field. It is obvious that the difficulty of this integrative task will vary according to the amounts of psychic tension and psychic energy that are bound in the various subsidiary goals and motor mechanisms."[7]

It is not without significance that French's bibliography includes not only wide reference to the work of Freud but also to that of Köhler, Lewin, Tolman, and Hull.

Lest it be thought, however, that the lions and the lambs have lain down together with a perfect serenity, Lewin's recent reply (28) to various of French's criticisms of topological psychology should be mentioned. Lewin points out that topological psychology has developed on an empirical basis as has psychoanalytic theory but that topological psychology has the following scientific advantages: first, a higher level of aspiration with regard to concepts; secondly, a "greater readiness to face the logical consequences of a theory without explaining non-fitting cases as exceptions . . . "; thirdly, stricter requirements regarding the proof of a theory; and finally, greater attention to the differences between historical and ahistorical questions.

It has been the purpose of this section on "critical discussions" to indicate concretely the beginnings of a trend in the literature toward a consolidation of the aims and theories of psychoanalysis and experimental psychology and the important

[7] pp. 245-246.

existing differences between them. The papers selected to illustrate this trend are only a sampling from an expanding literature.[8] Quotations from the work of both academic psychologists
and psychoanalysts were given in order to demonstrate the
reciprocal character of the "revision" in progress.

(2) Investigations of the "Influence of Emotions on
Memory"[9]

On the whole, "classical" experiments conducted by psychologists in the field of memory led to highly abstract laws
of memory functioning. Precisely because these abstract laws
bore so minimal a relation to the everyday function of memory,
the need for exploring the so-called "interfering factors" was
soon made apparent. Thus, there existed for a time an enthusiastic interest in phenomena labelled "retroactive inhibition",[10] "reminiscence", the effects of "set" and "context", and
so forth. This developing interest in "additional factors" in
memory functioning was given impetus by what appears now
to have been a serious misunderstanding and misapplication
of the Freudian theory of forgetting. Experimenters working in
this field assumed that Freud had believed quite literally that
" . . . we tend to forget the unpleasant" and so they proceeded
to set up experiments that completely disregarded the specific meaning of this expression in Freudian usage and certainly
its implications regarding unconscious psychological processes.
Thus, a host of vaguely "emotional" influences on memory were
investigated either as isolated curiosa or with the aim of prov-
ing or disproving the Freudian memory theory. Such terms

[8] Recent papers such as those of Kardiner (23) and Landis (25) further illustrate this general point. An excellent example of the impact of organismic
philosophy generally, and of Gestalt psychology in particular, on the study of
personality is Angyal's recent book (4) in which the stress is on theoretical
systematization. Equally organismic but closer to experimental and clinical
methods is the pioneering work at the Harvard Psychological Clinic, brought
together in Murray's suggestive account (33) of the results of cooperative experiments and clinical investigations.

[9] The most complete critical discussion of this work is that by Rapaport. (38).

[10] This specific phenomenon has been discussed recently by Edwards (13), in
a critical "restatement of the problem" of the retention of affective experiences.

as "hedonic", "affective", "pleasant-unpleasant", "liked-disliked" were used to indicate the nature of the influencing factor.

In one group of these experiments word-lists were the stock-in-trade. The subject was asked to learn them and the influence of the emotional factor on this learning was investigated either by introducing "pleasant" (P), "unpleasant" (U) or "indifferent" (I) sensory stimuli, or by presenting words which held P, U, or I connotations for a given subject. A host of such experiments were conducted; some were devoted to the development of rigid controls of such factors as length of list, recency, primacy, and so on. Others ventured into an investigation of the many possible variations of experimental set-up. Thus a great number of experiments studied delayed versus immediate recall; others, the problem of "overlearning" versus incidental memory; still others, the effects of age, sex, and intelligence on the learning of word-lists. This enumeration gives only the merest hint of the extent to which this type of experiment was developed.

In an effort to reduce the artificiality of the word-list learning experiments, other investigators used instead the recall of P, U, and I life experiences. In this series, too, there were meticulous controls attempted of the same type as those mentioned in connection with the word-list experiments.

Further efforts to study the "influence of emotions on memory" took the form of association experiments which used words with P, U, and I "feeling-tones". In addition to noting the reaction-time and the quality of the reaction to a given word, some of these studies included a reproduction experiment in which the subject was asked to repeat his previous reactions.

Although in all of these experiments the essential criterion for the "influence" of the emotional factor was the amount of material retained, there was some recognition of the importance of qualitative analyses. Instances of such qualitative analyses are the study of the course of the recall in reproduction, the analysis of the reaction word in the association experiments, and the study of the role of "context" and "set". Yet these qualitative findings were, for the most part, considered incidental and only subsidiary to the quantitative results.

Emphasis has been placed on the qualitative aspect of the experimental results only in a very few experiments. Rapaport (38) has selected as representative of these a study by Flanagan (17), two studies by Sharp (42) (43) and one by Diven (12). These studies in their implications pertained more directly to the Freudian theory of memory than any others.

Flanagan's investigation and Sharp's first study used paired nonsense syllables which when read together had a socially unacceptable or sexual meaning. They discovered, in addition to a quantitative impairment of the learning of these nonsense syllables as compared with the learning of innocuous pairs, a number of significant methods used by their subjects to circumvent the pronouncing of tabooed expressions. The subject would often misunderstand or distort the word formed by the paired syllables; sometimes he would condense them, utter them quickly or even forget them entirely. Both authors pointed out the similarities of these methods to the "Freudian mechanisms". However, they did not make it clear whether these techniques were adopted consciously and deliberately or whether they were adopted without the subject's being directly aware of the techniques themselves or their purpose. Despite this lack, the experimental results themselves are striking and significant.

In Sharp's second study the subjects were psychiatric patients. Sharp selected from their case-histories various nouns and adjectives directly related to their focal problems. The patients were then asked to learn lists of words among which were the "critical" nouns and adjectives selected from the case-history. Here again, Sharp found "mechanisms" similar to those described by Freud.

Diven, in an exceedingly sophisticated experimental study, used a series of stimulus words in which a pair of words recurred several times. In one series of experiments, called "con-

ditioning sessions", an experimental "trauma" was imposed on
the subject by giving him an electric shock simultaneous with
the second word of the recurring pair. The subject was then
asked to recall the stimulus words; this was followed by a "de-
conditioning session" in which no shocks were administered
and after which the subject was again asked to recall the stimulus words. There were several supplementary techniques used
and Diven presents a mass of detailed experimental results, in
the analysis of which he differentiates subjects who became
aware of the significance of the critical stimuli from those who
did not. This presentation will be restricted, however, to a
brief statement of the general results and of their significance
for the present problem. Diven found a "completely reliable"
increase in the average number of words recalled after "de-
conditioning" over that recalled before. He adduces evidence,
from his findings for "primary and secondary displacement",
for "dynamic repression" and for the "reactivation of a repressed complex". His data suggest a "relatively greater
strength of unconsciously integrated complexes".

This brief account of experimental investigations of the "influence of emotions on memory" has included the double aim
of demonstrating the numerous blind alleys to which over-
ambitious precision in memory experiments has led, and yet
the beginnings of "translatability" from the results of experiments to those of clinical investigations. In addition, it has
been shown that a hasty and superficial application of Freudian
theory to the construction or interpretation of an experiment
cannot but delay the ultimate integration of psychoanalytic
and experimental findings.

(3) Experiments Using Hypnosis

It is the aim of this discussion to present a few experiments
which have used hypnosis as a research tool and which have
direct implications for the present research. It will be seen
that this application of hypnosis to the problems of psychology,
particularly in recent experiments, promises some solution to
the dilemma of "vitality of material versus precision of method";

for the strong affective relationship between experimenter and the hypnotic subject makes possible the creation of psychological phenomena of significantly greater strength than those produced by the usual laboratory methods. This does not mean, however, that experimenters using hypnosis have always availed themselves of its great potentialities; many have used hypnosis in precisely the same artificial, rigid manner criticized in several of the previously discussed experiments on memory-function. Other investigators utilizing hypnosis have attempted to study the importance of "meaningful" versus "non-meaningful" material in work on hypnotic hypermnesia. Although there is still some debate on this question, one study by Stalnaker and Riddle (44) and another by White, Fox, and Harris (48) indicate the probability that earlier negative findings resulted from the use of meaningless material, thus precluding a creative reproduction. In contrast to the essentially qualitative analyses in the present research, both of these studies emphasized the quantitative differences between the normal and hypnotic recall of meaningful material.

The fact that certain acts may occur without awareness of their motivation had been demonstrated frequently by clinicians in the phenomenon of post-hypnotic suggestion. Erickson (15) brought this phenomenon into a close relation with psychoanalytic theory by his striking experiments on the "psychopathology of everyday life" in which he induced various socially unacceptable attitudes in his subjects during hypnosis, with the result that these attitudes came to expression during the subsequent normal state in the disguised form of slips of the tongue and parapraxes.

Young (50) discusses M. M. White's experiment (47) on "inhibition as a factor in recall" as a partial verification of the Freudian theory of repression, on the basis that White found a longer reaction-time to unpleasant words than to pleasant words in the hypnotic state. Although this finding is of interest, its relation to the Freudian theory of repression can be granted only by accepting a superficial understanding of this theory.

The problem of hypnotic regression is relevant here inasmuch as an attempt was made in the present research to reestablish a "tension system" several months after it had been induced in hypnosis. Although Platonow (36) has published extensively on the genuineness of this phenomenon, and although Erickson (14) has expressed the belief that this is the " . . . best and most promising aproach to date to one of the most significant . . . problems", Young (50) is not satisfied with the existing evidence and suggests the possibility that hypnotic regression may be simply an artifact.

Although the present research does not deal directly with the hypnotic production of "complexes", or of "experimental neuroses", brief mention should be made of the work in this field for two reasons: first, because in this area far more than in our own experiments there has been the most clear-cut attempt to incorporate *both* "vitality" and "precision"; and secondly, because any extension of the present experiments would of necessity need to take many cues from these investigations. The pioneering investigations into the "nature of human conflicts" were conducted by the Russian psychologist, A. R. Luria (30). He suggested to deeply hypnotized subjects experiences of such a nature as to result in a significant affective disturbance which, though rendered amnesic, would bring about discernible symptoms in the normal state. In both normal and hypnotic states, word-association tests were given; these were accompanied by meticulous measures of voluntary and involuntary motor responses. Clear evidence for the affective disturbance was found. Further, hypnotic psychotherapy was used to remove the conflict and this was proven efficacious by a readministration of the association tests and the measures of motor response. Luria's work, thus, was an attempt to demonstrate experimentally the operation of what has sometimes been called clinically an "unconscious complex".[11]

---

[11] Other investigations of this sort, which followed Luria's general mode of attack, have been summarized by P. C. Young (50).

(4) The Work of Lewin and Students

This group of experiments has been selected for discussion both because it provides part of the direct setting for the experiments to be described, and because the investigations of Lewin and his followers come closer to a systematic[12] synthesis of vitality and sound methodology than those of any other theoretical approach of academic psychology. Inasmuch as most of the early experiments by his students have been summarized by Lewin (26), this presentation will be limited to a sampling of the kinds of problems attacked by this group, the evidences for recent attempts at a rapprochement with psychoanalytic theory, and finally the precise contributions of these experiments to the formulation of the present problem.

Under the heading, "general laws of psychological systems", Lewin (26) includes the study of the formation of "tension systems" as the result of a "need", a "purpose", or an "intention". It is this area, particularly the work of Zeigarnik, with which the present research is directly concerned; a detailed discussion will be given of several pertinent investigations. Still under this general heading, Lewin discusses the experiments on "substitution", that is the " . . . question of the discharge of the psychical systems through substitute or compensatory activities . . . "[13] This problem is considered as the experimental analogue to the problem of "sublimation" in Freudian theory. Other studies in this sub-grouping include investigations of "level of aspiration" and "physical satiation".

Lewin includes also the problems of "general topology and dynamics" (for example, anger, as a dynamic problem) and problems of "reality and unreality". The implications of the latter for psychopathology are many; it will probably be one of the most important fields for cooperative research. A recent attempt—not experimental—to apply this concept to problems raised by psychoanalysts is that by MacKinnon (31); he gives a "topological analysis of anxiety" in terms of the simultaneous

[12] This is in contrast with important single experiments, not conceived within a given theoretical system, such as the work of Luria (30) previously discussed.
[13] p. 247.

and contradictory distortions on the levels of "positive and
negative unreality".

Yet another attempt to find a common ground conceptually
is that by French (19). In his discussion of dreams as a means
" . . . of studying the subjective factors in structuralization of
the field" he reports two consecutive dreams from a single
patient and says:

> "Different parts of the two dreams could be shown
> to be merely different ways of dealing with this one
> fundamental problem comparable to the changes in
> the practical grasp of the experimental situation
> achieved . . . by Köhler's monkeys. Just as Köhler's
> monkey is at first baffled by the problem of getting
> a banana just out of its reach . . . so the dream at-
> tempts first one method and then another of prac-
> tically grasping and reacting to the problem pre-
> sented by conflicting emotional urges . . . "[14]

Although this research is, at its present stage, concerned
only incidentally with the problem of "regression", a recent
major study by Barker, Dembo, and Lewin on "frustration and
regression" (5) will be considered here in some detail because
it is one of the best examples of an attempt to attack experimentally a problem " . . . at the intersection of historical and
systematic questions". It shows clearly both the strong and
weak aspects of a transitional investigation.

The authors begin with a discussion of the loose usage to
which the term "regression" has been subject, and they point
out Freud's recognition of the need for a conceptual refinement
of the term. There is included then a fairly detailed critique
of "regression" as understood by the psychoanalyst, and a distinction is drawn between "retrogression" regarded as a re-
instatement of an earlier behavior pattern and "regression" as
discussed in terms of a "de-differentiation" and "primitiviza-
tion" of the person. The experiment is concerned thus with
the concept, "regression".

[14] p. 17.

Using the most advanced experimental techniques in child psychology, the investigators constructed an elaborate laboratory situation: thirty pre-school children were first observed in a "free play situation" and later in a "frustrating situation" where a number of more attractive toys had been added but rendered inaccessible by replacing one of the walls of the room by an impregnable wire-net, through which the toys could be seen but not reached. Interest in the new toys was guaranteed by permitting the child to play with them for a little while before letting down the wire-net between the child and the toys. The criterion used for determining the resulting "regression" was the extent to which the productivity of the child, with the accessible toys, decreased in this frustrating situation as compared with the previous free play situation. A careful scale of "constructiveness" was developed, and it was found that "a background of frustration decreases the average constructiveness of play with accessible toys . . . by an amount equivalent to 17.3 months of mental age".[15] Other suggestive results are offered, and it is stated that "probably different factors were important for different subjects".[16]

This study is perhaps one of the best examples of the "transitional experiment". No one could say that its problem is pedantic or sterile. Equally, it could not be said that the methods used were loose or "literary". Yet one cannot feel that in this type of experiment lies the final solution to the problem of combining "vitality" and "precision", although there can be little question that it is one of the most promising approaches yet devised by experimental psychologists. The inadequacies of such experiments are perhaps related to their tremendous refinement and differentiation of small areas of great problems which themselves are not yet clearly comprehended even in a gross manner. In a sense, it may be that the precision of such experiments has outgrown the present grasp of the underlying problems, and this fact may create a

[15] p. 207.
[16] p. 216.

feeling in the reader that there is "too much talk about too little". Perhaps the course of experimentation should proceed from the opposite direction with attempts to achieve some feeling for the gross total pattern of the "whole elephant" before proceeding with histological investigations of the tissues of his ear. There can be no question, for example, but that the Freudian theory of regression includes phenomena of a magnitude and depth not within the scope of this investigation. This is not to say that the observed phenomena in this study are unimportant or invalid, but that the differences between these phenomena and the monumental changes in a clinically observed regression must not be underestimated, nor must they be regarded as the inevitable price of scientific investigation. It may be that the experimentalist will be enabled to come closer even than he has to the study of central rather than peripheral phenomena.

Rapaport (39), in a critical discussion of "Freudian mechanisms and frustration" says:

> "The similarity of the phenomena observed in frustration experiments to the Freudian mechanisms is obvious. The gravest danger in dealing with them lies in the possibility that one may lose sight of the fact that our knowledge about them has been gathered in a methodologically basically different way than knowledge of the Freudian mechanisms. The Freudian mechanisms reflect vicissitudes of instinctual needs inferred from historical investigations. The reactions to frustration in the frustration experiments are ahistorically established dynamics of a field situation out of which no conclusion as to the genetic relation between frustration and its sequelae should be drawn."

Although these comments were made specifically with regard to frustration experiments, the same might be said of the experimental investigation of any psychoanalytic concept. Thus the evaluation of the experiments on "repression" now to be considered should be based at least partly on the above considerations.

A study by Gould (21), called "An Experimental Investigation of Repression" was reported in part at a meeting of topological psychologists. She described her procedures as follows:

> "The experimental technique creates a conflict in a context which is potentially a threat to the self-esteem or ego of the individual. The subject is presented with two tasks from which he must choose one to perform. He is told that the nature of his choice will reveal a particular personality characteristic. Regardless of his choice, however, he is given a pre-arranged personality evaluation. Each subject is presented with six (6) choice situations and is given six (6) personality comments after each of these choices, three (3) positive and three (3) negative."[17]

It was expected that the behavior of the subject in response to the comments, as well as the characteristics of the recall of both tasks and comments, would provide a means for investigating various nuclear problems regarding the repression process, such as the criteria for repression, the specific role of the emotional factor in repression, the determining factor that dictates repression as a 'path out of conflict' and so on. In analyzing her results, Gould places more emphasis on the qualitative than on the quantitative findings; she concludes "presumptive evidence for repression" and offers a ". . . two-fold hypothesis concerning the psychodynamics of repression . . .":

> "(1) The level of emotional tension . . . determines the extent of possible recall of that situation; (2) the specific motivational pattern operating at the time selectively determines, within the range set by the tension level, what aspects of the situation will be re-

[17] p. 40.

> called. A high level of tension makes repression possible. . . . In conjunction with a high level of tension, certain motivational factors determine that those aspects of the situation which arouse anxiety and tension, shall . . . suffer most in recall."

In addition, quantitative results are cited to give supportive evidence that repression was actually created by the experiments. For example, the comments, though fewer in number, are forgotten relatively more often than the tasks; also, the tasks associated with U-comments are forgotten more often than tasks associated with P-comments, and a U-task initially forgotten and spontaneously recalled during the interview is often accompanied by intense affect toward the task.

Like the frustration-regression experiment at Iowa, Gould's investigation is transitional and therefore relevant to the present research. It, again, attempts to apply a more rigorous method to the study of a dynamic concept. Yet, precisely because it is so restricted in its content, it is difficult to accept it as a bonafide relative of Freud's description of repression. It may be that the "level" of the need or striving evoked by this experiment is quite different from the type of striving or wish that is repressed in everyday life. Even though one may grant the possibility that *similar* mechanisms may be involved, it is of little use to call the phenomena produced experimentally, "repression" until one can demonstrate a more organic relationship between the experimental and the clinical phenomena. In Erickson's experimental demonstration of the psychopathology of everyday life (15) for instance, this organic relation exists so obviously that no one would question its relevance to the psychoanalytic theory of parapraxes; yet even this experiment added nothing to its conceptual refinement. It is clear thus that the tremendous complexity of psychoanalytic concepts is not to be underestimated and that there is perhaps more to be lost than gained by an easy identification of experimental processes with the various Freudian concepts: in this instance with the concept of repression.

Although Zeigarnik (51) dealt only incidentally with the problem of repression, her experiments and those of Ovsiankina (34) will be discussed here because they provided techniques which have been applied to many different kinds of experiments, some of which have stated explicitly that their purpose was to study the process of repression with experimental methods. The present research has adapted the Zeigarnik technique for the exploration of the vicissitudes of "tension systems" originated in normal and hypnotic states.

Zeigarnik, in her classic experiments, gave a series of eighteen to twenty simple tasks to a number of subjects, allowing them to complete only half of the tasks and interrupting the other half before the subject was able to finish. The subject was then asked to recall the tasks; Zeigarnik found a 90 per cent mean advantage in recall of the interrupted over the completed tasks. This advantage was held to be an indication of the existence of a "quasi-need" to complete the interrupted task, and thus experimental corroboration of the Lewinian theory of "tension systems" was provided. Numerous control experiments were introduced to show that the undischarged "tension system" and not some other factor was responsible for the results. This material has been summarized adequately and frequently in the reports of subsequent experiments which have stemmed from the work of Zeigarnik and Ovsiankina, who demonstrated the same essential point by observing the high per cent of resumptions of interrupted tasks. Refinements of technique and elaboration of problems inherent in the use of the "Zeigarnik technique" have expanded the literature to the point that there now exists an extensive bibliography of experiments using the method of interrupted tasks. Investigations by Pachauri (35), Marrow (32), Katz (24), Schlote (41) and others generally substantiated Zeigarnik's findings.

Recently, a number of experimenters have become interested in radically varying the conditions of the Zeigarnik experiment in order to investigate the different ways in which a "tension system" may be structured, and in some instances to investigate the relation of such differences to the psychoanalytic concept of repression. Rosenzweig (40) has reported an experiment in which every subject was given a number of jig-saw puzzles to do; the experimenter let the subject complete only half of the puzzles. However, he divided his subjects into two groups presenting the puzzles as an intelligence test to one group and in an informal spirit to the other. Those subjects who regarded the experiment as a test tended to favor the finished puzzles in recall, while those who had done the puzzles informally tended to recall the unfinished puzzles more frequently. In a subsequent discussion Rosenzweig draws a distinction between what he calls "need-persistive" and "ego-defensive" reactions to frustration, and concludes that in this experiment the members of the informal group were under little tension and their interest was centered on the task ("need-persistive" reaction), while those in the formal group were under considerable tension and incompletion meant the evocation of feelings of failure ("ego-defensive" reaction). Rosenzweig proposes these "two fundamental types" of reaction as a framework for most of the psychoanalytic mechanisms and in this instance calls his experiment, therefore, an "experiment on repression".

Although Rosenzweig's study is still a relatively crude approach to the delicate and subtle character of the process of repression as described by Freud, its importance in raising certain focal problems has been overlooked in the literature. For example, Adler and Kounin (2), in a recent paper reviewing the general status of the problem of interrupted tasks, cited Rosenzweig's experiment as one of the few instances of "contradictory evidence" on the question of whether interrupted tasks are better retained than completed ones. They say:

> "The authors believe that the discrepancies between Rosenzweig's data and those of others are due to his

use of a 'success and failure' rather than an interruption technique."[18]

Thus Rosenzweig's results are regarded as due to a technical innovation and therefore of trifling significance. If, instead, Rosenzweig's data were seen as broadening and developing the problem rather than as "contradicting" Zeigarnik's findings, the existing "island-character" of various isolated researches would tend to be somewhat neutralized. Rosenzweig hints at the possible integrative value of his experiment in his establishment of the "need-persistive" versus "ego-defensive" reaction types. This dichotomy is perhaps too restricted, however, and serves to obscure the possibility, suggested by Rapaport, (38) of the existence of an emotional hierarchy of highly differentiated gradations which shade from relatively peripheral needs or strivings to more central ones. Although Lewin (27) has hinted at such a stratification in his discussion of the "topology of the person", particularly in his description of the "inner-personal strata", his distinction between "central" and "peripheral" inner-personal strata seems still decidedly in the blue-print state. J. D. Frank (18) has recently pointed out the need for a greater clarification of Lewin's "representation of the person". Such a development would be precluded by considering the results of the Rosenzweig experiment "contradictory" to those of the Zeignarik experiment. The relevance of these theoretical considerations regarding allied problems to the findings of the present research will be considered in detail in the discussion following the presentation of the experiments themselves.

Adler (1) has reported other pertinent studies in a paper entitled, "The Experimental Production of Repression."[19] In

[18] p. 256.

[19] Adler has appended a footnote to the title of his paper, suggesting that the phenomena described are significantly different from repression in the Freudian sense and should more properly be called "suppression". However, this qualifying statement was apparently an after-thought; the body of the report uses the term "repression" throughout.

one study conducted by Blumberg, the subject was given six-teen jig-saw puzzles to put together; half were bright and sharply defined, the other half, dull and unclear. All were in-terrupted. The subject was told that this was an intelligence test and that he would be rated. After each interruption of an easy puzzle, the subject was told he was doing better than average; after interruption on the harder ones, he was told his performance was poorer than average. When all sixteen puz-zles had been administered, the experimenter asked for recall and found that those who did not accept the experimenter's judgment of failure and who felt they could have done better recalled more failure-puzzles than successes, while those who experienced real failure recalled more success-puzzles than failures. Blumberg concludes that in this second group " . . . the experience of failure led to an inability to recall the failed activity, i.e., to repression."[20] A second experiment, conducted by Adler and reported in this same paper, employs a procedure with adults used by Wright (49) to study altruism in children. The subject must decide which of two tasks (one judged pleas-ant and the other unpleasant) to do himself and which to leave for a stranger to do. The assumption was that if the "selfish" decisions actually produced guilt then perhaps there should be some difficulty in recalling those tasks related to the "selfish" choices. Adler's preliminary results indicate that in the recall, the "selfish" choices *are* forgotten more frequently than the "generous" ones. As the result of an attempt to "bring back" the forgotten items by a removal of guilt, Adler found some evidence that this guilt removal does permit a freer return of memory for the "selfish" choices in an additional recall period. This increase was compared with the character of the recall in a "guilty" group for which the experimenter made no at-tempt to remove the guilt and which, accordingly, recalled fewer "selfish" choices in the additional recall.

   Although there can be little doubt that the phenomena des-cribed in all of these "repression" experiments are genuine and

[20] p. 25.

possess an independent validity, it must again be emphasized in conclusion that their relevance to the phenomena designated by the Freudian term will not be clear until the specific relationships of the central and peripheral "inner-personal strata" to each other and to Freudian "unconscious drives" are worked out.

III. *Accounts of the Experiments*

Before proceeding to the experimental accounts, several methodological and technical problems should be mentioned. The entire series of experiments uses the method of systematic variation with few subjects rather than that of literal repetitions with large numbers. Quite apart from the fact that Fisher (16) and others have recognized the value of using qualitative methods to increase the sensitiveness of an experiment, this approach is dictated by the high degree of selection and the intensive training of subjects necessary for work with hypnosis. For example, it is not at all unusual to find that from a group of twenty volunteers, one can use only one or two subjects for certain kinds of experiments. When these are selected on the basis of their reactions in a group hypnosis, the "weeding-out" process is fairly simple. However, when these rare subjects must be found by trial-and-error in individual hypnosis, the practical problem is far more serious. Thus, the statistical treatment of the data is extremely crude inasmuch as the samples are necessarily so small. However, it has been possible to deal intensively with qualitative data and with some trends in the quantitative data.

It was mentioned in the section on background material that the work of Zeigarnik (51) provides the direct antecedents of these investigations. It will be recalled that Zeigarnik found that, in general, if a person is given a number of tasks and permitted to complete only half of them, he will recall the interrupted tasks significantly better than those completed, thus revealing the persistence of a "tension system" related to the "quasi-need" to complete the interrupted task. It was found also that subjects have a strong wish to resume tasks that have been interrupted. A good hypnotic subject, preferably one who has been developed by systematic training to the point of deepest "somnambulism", can be made to forget not only having been interrupted in certain tasks but even having seen the task materials. Thus, it has been possible to initiate the investigation of the following problems: (1) What is the influence on behavior in the normal state of a "tension system" created in hypnosis, and conversely, the influence on behavior in the hypnotic state of a "tension system" created in the normal state? (2) Can a "tension system" created in one state (normal or hypnotic) be discharged in the other? (3) What is the relationship between the spontaneous needs set into operation by the hypnosis itself and the experimentally induced quasi-needs? (4) Is it possible by a technique of hypnotic "regression" to re-create a "tension system" after a period during which, under Zeigarnik's conditions, it would have completely disintegrated? (5) What is the relation of reality levels in hypnosis to those in the normal state?

This list by no means exhausts the theoretical possibilities for exploring the structure and the fate of "tension systems" in normal and hypnotic states. It simply offers a glimpse of the kind of problem for which this general approach seems best suited.

(1) The Influence on the Normal State of a "Tension System" Created in Hypnosis

Statement of the Problem: The results of both psychoanalytic and hypnotic clinical investigations have suggested that frequently behavior is determined by needs, strivings, or goals of which the individual has no direct awareness; the aim of this experiment was to apply a more standardized technique, developed by an experimental psychologist, to the study of this problem. If it could be shown that a "tension system" created in hypnosis has observable effects on the behavior in the normal state when the subject has amnesia for the origin of the "tension system", then perhaps this would open a path to the systematic exploration of "unconscious mechanisms".

Subjects: This problem was explored on three separate occasions: twice with the same subject, Alice A., using radically different techniques each time and once with Barbara B., essentially a confirmation of the first experiment with Alice A. Alice A. is a nurse, aged twenty-six, who had a year of psychiatric training but had never seen any hypnosis. She is a top-notch subject, one of the upper 5 per cent of the population. From the first, she showed most of the extreme hypnotic phenomena. Barbara B. is a high school senior, aged seventeen; she is an attractive, somewhat frivolous youngster and has never read a book on psychology. She had seen hypnosis once on the stage and had been skeptical of it. Her response to hypnosis was immediately deep; she showed a good amnesia after the first session and was subsequently developed into a somnambulistic subject.

Procedure with Alice A: In order to secure the most reliable kind of hypnosis, Alice A. was trained in a number of preliminary sessions, each of which served to familiarize her with the general phenomena of the hypnotic state. For example, Alice A. expressed the belief that hypnosis is essentially a passive lethargic state resembling sleep and that one cannot be in hypnosis with his eyes open. Therefore, the fact that she could open her eyes and yet remain in a deep "trance" was proved to her satisfaction when, with her eyes open, she experienced functional paralysis of her legs at the suggestion of the experimenter. Another session was designed to let Alice A. experience actively "doing things" in hypnosis without disrupting the "trance". Although this may seem an overcautious and laborious procedure, it seemed to us preferable to spend considerable time in training a subject than to introduce a subject to a critical situation and risk ruining the experiment.

When it appeared that the preliminary training period had taken into account most of such possible unevenness in Alice A.'s response to hypnosis, the experiments were begun. Alice was first asked in the *normal* state to select the preferred one of a pair of tasks in ten pairs.[21] She was shown each task and told:

[21] The ten pairs of tasks are listed; many were adapted from Zeigarnik (51) and Marrow (32): (See Table V, p. 252 for order of task presentation).

1. Copy a geometrical design (P) / or 2. Construct a geometrical figure with match-sticks.

"I'm going to show you a number of tasks and I'd like you to tell me which one of two you'd rather do. I don't want you to do them, but just tell me which you *would* prefer."

When Alice A. had given all of her preferences in the normal state, she was deeply hypnotized and amnesia for these choices was induced. Still in hypnosis, she was given the twenty tasks to do; half were interrupted and half completed with an equal number of preferred tasks interrupted and completed.[22] She was then brought out of hypnosis with complete amnesia both for her original preferences in the normal state and for her task performance in the hypnotic state. Now, back in the normal state, she was again asked which of each pair of tasks she preferred.[23]

3. Cut out and color a tulip / or 4. Cut out sport outfit in fashion magazine (P).
5. Arrange scrambled panels of cartoon-strip to make joke / or 6. Put manikin profile together (P).
7. Jig-saw puzzle / or 8. Copy block design (P).
9. Simple cross-word puzzle (P) / or 10. Put together cut-up proverbs to make sense.
11. Cut design out of paper by folding / or 12. Fill in blanks in sentences (P).
13. Number puzzle (P) / or 14. Simple arithmetic problems.
15. Fill ellipses with crosses (P) / or 16. Complete a series of squares.
17. Find an actor, a city, a state, and a body of water starting with same letter / or 18. Build a sentence from the words: crowd, hatred, wire, table (P).
19. Draw plan of hospital grounds (P) / or 20. Draw plan of school grounds. ("P" means preferred task)

[22] See Table V (p. 252) for order of presentation.

[23] For practical reasons we selected shifts in task-preference as a means of studying the formation and vicissitudes of the "tension systems". Clearly, we could not ask for recall in the normal state which followed her task performance in hypnosis because she had amnesia for the entire experience. Another possibility might have been to use task-resumption as a means of checking the state of the evidenced tension systems; this was ruled out by the experimental plan which included the necessity to maintain the "tension system" rather than to discharge it by allowing the subject to complete the tasks. We recognize that the use of shifts in task preference introduces a host of unexplored problems on the determinants of "what is preferred" and actually our results with control groups who were not hypnotized at any time suggests that the dynamics of "preference" are somewhat different from those of recall or resumption. In order to properly evaluate our tentative findings, it would be necessary to conduct an independent study of task-preference.

Results with Alice A: Two reversals of preference occurred: whereas in her original choices in the normal state Alice A. had preferred the cross-word puzzle task (9) to putting together the proverbs (10), her preference was now reversed; a similar reversal took place between tasks (19) and (20). It is apparent that if no change in the "valence" of the tasks had taken place, she would have preferred five interrupted and five completed tasks, inasmuch as five preferred tasks were interrupted and five were completed. Her "preference-quotient" would then have been 5/5 or 1.0. Instead, she preferred seven completed tasks and three interrupted tasks, yielding a "preference-quotient" of .42 and indicating a need either to avoid the interrupted tasks or to repeat the completed tasks.

Procedure with Barbara B.:   The procedure here was essentially a repetition of the experiment on Alice A. The tasks used were different[24] and the Zeigarnik experiment in hypnosis was not conducted on the same day that the original preferences were made. Aside from these two deviations, the experiment with Barbara B. was carried out in precisely the same manner as that with Alice A.

Results with Barbara B.:   Here again, the preference-shift in the direction of the completed tasks appeared *after* Barbara was brought out of hypnosis with amnesia for having done twenty tasks and completing only half of them, in hypnosis. In this normal state, then, following the Zeigarnik experiment in hypnosis, she preferred three interrupted tasks and seven completed tasks. This clearly shows that two tasks previously

[24] These ten pairs of tasks were also adapted from several sources as indicated in the listing for the experiment with Alice A.:
1. Do a simple multiplication (P) / or 2. Write an old nursery rhyme.
3. Model a clay animal / or 4. Draw a vase (P).
5. Make a mosaic design (P) / or 6. String beads.
7. Fill a paper with crosses / or 8. Copy a paragraph (P).
9. Connect scattered numbers from 1-20 (P) / or 10. Maze puzzle.
11. Jig-saw puzzle / or 12. Write 12 cities or states starting with 3 different letters, 4 in each group (P).
13. Underline l's and n's in a paragraph (P) / or 14. Count crosses on a page.
15. Draw a girl / or 16. Make design with colored paper (P).
17. Sorting task (P) / or 18. Peg construction.
19. Punch holes / or 20. Outline a star (P).

"preferred", which were interrupted during the experiment, have now become "non-preferred"; thus the theoretical quotient of 1.0 which would result had the preferences undergone no change is reduced to 3/7 or .42, just as in the experiment with Alice A., indicating again either a wish to avoid the interrupted or to repeat the completed tasks.

Use of a second technique with Alice A.: The question was raised that perhaps even the neutral tasks given Alice A. in the first experiment were variable with regard to their attractiveness; although the *shift* in task-preference toward the completed tasks made this consideration appear less significant, it was thought worthwhile to explore the same problem, using nonsense syllables. This experiment was conducted five months after the first experiment with Alice A.

Procedure: The technique used here was adapted from an unpublished study by K. B. Watson (46) carried out under the direction of Adams: Alice A. in a state of deep hypnosis was given a sheet of paper with the lines numbered from one to twenty, and with a nonsense syllable at the top. She was given the general instruction for the whole period to copy the nonsense syllable on each line of the page but was interrupted, of course, in half of the trials. The point of interruption was always somewhere between lines fifteen and twenty. She was given only one sheet at a time and did not know how many to expect; twenty syllables were used altogether.[25] Amnesia was induced for the experiment thus far and Alice A., still in hypnosis, was given the list of nonsense syllables and asked to choose the ten in order of preference that she would choose to copy if she were asked to copy some.

Results: She chose seven syllables that she had been allowed to complete and three that had been interrupted ("preference-quotient" is thus 3/7 or .42). She was asked to make these choices first in hypnosis in order to see whether the

---

[25] The nonsense syllables used in this experiment were the following: meev, jish, glet, crad, lerm, sark, goje, hool, fape, kise, roif, twic, theg, chuz, daux, bune, nowk, whab, dalm, krof. (See Table VI, p. 253 for specific order of presentation and syllables preferred in normal and hypnotic states).

preference for the completed tasks in the normal state after
the Zeigarnik experiment in hypnosis in the previous experiment might be because of the sudden transition from a hypnotic to a normal state. Apparently, this was not the reason
for the shift in preference. She was then brought back to the
normal state and asked her preferences. She still preferred
the completed tasks, though not so definitely as in the preceding hypnotic state: she chose four interrupted and six
completed tasks, yielding a "preference-quotient" of 4/6 or .66.
Thus, it appeared that this experiment using nonsense syllables
instead of semi-meaningful tasks substantiated the results of
the first two experiments. The preference for the *completed*
tasks after the Zeigarnik experiment was conducted in hypnosis seemed clear.

Discussion: On the basis of the Zeigarnik and Ovsiankina
experiments, the expectation had been that a "tension system"
created in hypnosis would behave very much like a "tension system" created in the normal state, the only difference being that
in hypnosis, it would be possible to render the origin of the
"tension system" inaccessible to the direct awareness of the
subject. Thus, it had been thought that in the normal state
directly following the Zeigarnik experiment in hypnosis the
subject would prefer more interrupted than completed tasks.
Precisely the opposite occurred. In each of the three experiments, the subject in the normal state preferred the completed tasks after the experiment and in one case preferred
the C-tasks in hypnosis directly after it. This fact could
mean one of three things: first, perhaps there was no "tension
system" set up at all; secondly, if such a "tension system"
were set up it may have been disrupted by some intense intervening experience; and thirdly, it might have been created but
obscured by some other, more urgent motivating factor.

Zeigarnik (51) has described several situations in which
these three possibilities are illustrated. For example, she conducted experiments which showed that the completed tasks
have an advantage in recall if the experiment is conducted

while the subject is fatigued. The rationale given for this finding is the following, according to Pachauri (34):

> "There are, as it were, two forces at work in the U-C effect, the strain of U-tasks in virtue of unresolved urge, and the strain of C-tasks in virtue of accomplished *form*."[26]

That this hypothesis was unlikely was indicated by other data, derived from extensions of these experiments performed on the same day and described in the next section on the discharge of "tension systems". The second possibility, namely disruption by a violent intervening experience, seemed unlikely in view of the fact that the preference for the completed tasks was evident not only when there was a transition from the hypnotic to the normal states but also when preference was asked in the hypnotic state directly following the experiment.[27] Of course, it might be said that any subject in hypnosis is in an "excitable" state and thus would give a reduced value of U over C tasks. Other data, to be presented, seem to obviate this possibility as well. Yet another possibility was suggested by the fact that pre-knowledge of the content of the tasks has been shown to decrease the "Zeigarnik ratio". Although the subjects were made amnesic for their having first seen the tasks in the normal state, it might be argued that there was retained some sense of "familiarity" with the tasks and that, therefore, the preference-quotient was below 1.0, indicating a favoring of the completed tasks. However, it will be recalled that in the experiment employing nonsense syllables, Alice A. had never before seen the tasks.

Inasmuch as the first two hypotheses seemed unlikely, the third was tentatively adopted. This hypothesis, that the "quasi-need" created by the experiment to finish the tasks was "drowned out" by a more central need, was specifically formulated as follows: if the need to complete the interrupted task

[26] This argument will be again referred to in the final discussion.
[27] See account of experiment on Alice A., using nonsense syllables.

were imbedded in the more general need to please or literally obey the experimenter then the subject in hypnosis would regard the interruption as a prohibition, though it were given mildly; the wish to complete the interrupted tasks would thus be temporarily obscured because the subject would feel that he had failed to please the experimenter and had been "forbidden" to work on the uncompleted tasks. His preference for the completed tasks was thus regarded as a wish to avoid the "tabooed" activities. It was assumed that if this hypothesis were correct, a *severe* prohibition to continue with a task even in the normal state should have a roughly similar result. Accordingly, the usual Zeigarnik experiment with critical variations was conducted with two groups of college students *in the normal state.*

Control Experiments: In one group of college students the subjects were interrupted in a severe and slightly threatening manner, and in the other the interruptions were mild and friendly.[28] The subjects in both groups were asked for *both* recall and preference of the tasks after they had been permitted to complete half of the twenty[29] tasks and were interrupted in the other half.

Results of Control Experiments: In line with the prediction, the members of the "prohibitive group", like the hypnotic subjects, recalled and preferred more completed tasks than did the "mild group" (See Tables I and II).

Table I gives the results in the "mild group"; this group is probably more like Zeigarnik's original experimental group than is the "prohibitive group" (See Table II). Evidence for

[28] The exact wording of the interruption was varied somewhat to prevent a stereotyped interjection devoid of all affect. The basic structure, however, and the interruption in each group was constant. In the "prohibitive group" the interruption was given sternly and in a somewhat domineering manner: "Stop now! *Right away.* I don't want you to work on that any more at all!" or "That's all on that; you *must not* work on that any more!" In the mild group, the interruption was casual and friendly: "That's enough on that one, now. Let's do another." or "O.K., I see how you do that one. Now I'd like you to do this one."

[29] The tasks used in these experiments were the same as those used in the experiment with Barbara B. See footnote 24, p. 226.

this is the fact that the averages of the absolute numbers of unfinished (U) and completed (C) tasks recalled in the "mild group" so closely resemble Zeigarnik's figures. In Lewin's (26) account of Zeigarnik's experiment, the average of the U-tasks recalled is 6.8 and that of the C-tasks, 4.25 yielding a difference of 2.5. In the "mild group" the average number of U-tasks recalled is 6.0 and C-tasks, 3.8, yielding a comparable difference of 2.2. Also, the "arithmetic mean"[30] of the $\frac{RU}{RC}$-quotients (recalled-unfinished over recalled-completed) is 1.9 in Zeignarik's experiment and 1.8 in the "mild group" here, if two subjects, established as atypical prior to calculating averages, are excluded from the computations.

In decided contrast with these figures, Table II shows the results in the "prohibitive group". The average "recall-quotient" is 1.36. This figure shows thus only a 36 per cent advantage in recall for the interrupted tasks. This should be compared with the 80 per cent average advantage ($\frac{RU}{RC}=1.8$) for the interrupted tasks in the "mild" group and with the 90 per cent average advantages in Zeigarnik's group. The average number of unfinished and completed tasks recalled in the "prohibitive group" shows a similar difference. A comparison of the median figures in both groups again points in the same direction, although less sharply.

A similar trend is shown by a comparison of the "preference-quotients"[31] in Tables I and II. In the "mild group" the average quotient is .76, indicating some preference for the completed tasks. In the "prohibitive group" this preference for the completed tasks is more marked, the average quotient being .61. This difference is brought out far more sharply by

[30] Marrow (32) has shown that the averaging of these ratios by Zeigarnik was statistically illegitimate. If a comparison is made, however, of "corrected values" in both experiments, the results are still roughly comparable.

[31] It will be recalled that a "preference-quotient" of 1.0 indicates that the unfinished and completed tasks are preferred equally often, a quotient below 1.0, a preference for the completed tasks, and a quotient above 1.0, a preference for the unfinished tasks.

a comparison of the median "preference-quotients" in the two groups. In the "mild group", the median quotient is .80 while in the "prohibitive group", it is .42. Thus it seems clear that although both prefer the completed tasks directly after the experiment, this preference for the completed tasks is much stronger in the "prohibitive group".

TABLE I

Recall and Preference Quotients in "Mild" Control Group

Subject	Recall			Preference		
	RU	RC	$\frac{RU}{RC}$	PU	PC	$\frac{PU}{PC}$
1. R. M.	7	2	3.5	2	8	.25
2. C. F.	6	3	2.0	4	6	.66
3. B. C.	8	5	1.6	4	6	.66
4. V. N.	6	4	1.5	4	5	.80
5. J. B.	3	2	1.5	4	5	.80
6. H. M.	7	6	1.15	5	5	1.0
7. B. B.[32]	7	6	1.15	1	9	.11
8. K. M.	5	5	1.0	5	5	1.0
9. L. Y.[32]	3	6	.50	2	6	.33
Means:						
1. Including 2 atypical S's	5.7	4.3	1.6	3.4	6.1	.64
2. Excluding 2 atypical S's	6.0	3.8	1.8	4.0	5.7	.76
Medians:						
1. Including 2 atypical S's	6.0	5.0	1.5	4.0	6.0	.66
2. Excluding 2 atypical S's	6.0	4.0	1.5	4.0	5.0	.80

Note: Although the sum of PU and PC should equal 10 in each case, it is necessary in some cases to change the planned division of U- and C-tasks (e.g., when an S finishes a U-task too soon). Thus, such tasks are omitted.

[32] Atypical subjects.

TABLE II

Recall and Preference Quotients in "Prohibitive" Control
Group

Subject	Recall			Preference		
	RU	RC	$\frac{RU}{RC}$	PU	PC	$\frac{PU}{PC}$
1. M. I.	7	3	2.33	3	7	.42
2. G. P.	7	5	1.40	4	6	.66
3. C. F.	4	3	1.33	4	6	.66
4. M. R.	5	4	1.25	2	8	.25
5. D. T.	5	4	1.25	3	7	.42
6. P. R.	7	6	1.16	3	7	.42
7. J. M.	6	7	.85	6	4	1.50
Means	5.8	4.5	1.36	3.5	6.4	.61
Medians	8.0	4.0	1.25	3.0	7.0	.42

RU, number of uncompleted tasks recalled (up to 1st long
    pause).
RC, number of completed tasks recalled (up to 1st long
    pause).
$\frac{RU}{RC}$ ratio of uncompleted to completed tasks recalled: "Zeigarnik Quotient".
PU, number of uncompleted tasks preferred.
PC, number of completed tasks preferred.
$\frac{PU}{PC}$ ratio of uncompleted to completed tasks preferred.

Although the established *difference* between the "preference quotients" of the two groups is the point of greatest interest for the present problem, the fact that *both* groups show
a preference for the completed tasks raises a problem of considerable theoretical interest on the determinants of task-
preference.

Table III presents the most significant quantitative com-
parisons of the "mild" and "prohibitive" groups in these control experiments. It shows the greater advantage of the interrupted tasks (in recall and in preference) in the "mild group".
The percentages were derived from Tables I and II.

TABLE III

A Comparison of the Recalls and Preferences in the "Mild" and "Prohibitive" Control Groups

		Mild	Prohibitive
Per cent advantage of *Unfinished* tasks (recall)	Mean	80%	36%
	Median	50%	25%
Per cent advantage of *Completed* tasks (preference)	Mean	24%	39%
	Median	20%	58%

For example, the 80 per cent advantage in recall of the unfinished tasks in the "mild group" refers to the fact that the mean recall quotient in the "mild group" is 1.8 (see Table I). The higher those figures are the greater appears to be the "quasi-need" to finish the interrupted tasks. The other percentages were derived in the same way. Inasmuch as the completed tasks were preferred in both the "mild" and in the "prohibitive" groups, the only meaningful comparison is between the per cent advantages of each. Clearly, thus, a higher figure here means a greater advantage for the completed tasks and thus a lesser "quasi-need" to complete the interrupted tasks. Table III shows thus that in terms of recall the "mild group" shows the greater "quasi-need" to complete the unfinished tasks and also that the "mild group" prefers more interrupted tasks than does the "prohibitive group". The first of these two results is the more clear-cut.

The qualitative observations reinforce the quantitative trends. It was apparent from the relative lack of spontaneous talk in the "prohibitive group" that the severe interruption was quite different from the casual interruption in the "mild group". However, it was curious to note that only a few subjects admitted genuine irritation at the manner of interruption. Only one subject (M. R.) expressed herself rather vehemently regarding the interruption:

> *"You kept stopping me all the time . . . I like to finish what I start . . . when you'd interrupt me I'd be working hard enough that I really could be mad.*

I was annoyed. I don't see that it was necessary to be so terse." (This was all said in clear irritation, in a sullen manner.)

In this particular instance, the experimenter had noted *before* the end of the experiment that the character of the interruption had been especially severe and that this might influence the results. Actually M.R.'s "preference-quotient" was the lowest in the "prohibitive" group. In another instance (J. M.), an analysis of the interview provided a clue to the fact that hers was the only recall quotient below 1.0 in the "prohibitive group". When J. M. was asked about her conclusions regarding the interruption, she said: "I imagined it was surely timing and that it meant I was slow on those tasks. I guessed I did better when I finished."

Evidence of yet another sort comes from K. M.'s behavior. He came into the laboratory, looking bored and a trifle supercilious. His first comment in response to the first task was: "Oh, gosh, I don't see any point in that at all—everybody does the same thing, don't they?" After the second task, he said: "I'll just tell you what I would do and then I won't do it—O. K.? That's just as good, isn't it?" During the third task: "Aw shucks, I don't believe in this stuff, do you?" At this point, the prediction was made (and recorded) that there was little likelihood of there being any "tension system" set up in this subject. The experiment continued and K. M., an exceedingly intelligent, witty student continued to joke and to make light remarks about the experiment. He recalled five interrupted and five completed tasks (recall-quotient, 1.0); and he preferred five interrupted and five completed tasks (preference-quotient, 1.0). The prediction that there would be no "tension system" formed, was thus checked. This instance is of importance because it illustrates so clearly the need for more than a peripheral involvement in the creation of even a "quasi-need". These qualitative data could easily be duplicated by a number of other individual case records. However, they are a representative sampling.

Summary and Comment. Several experiments with hypnotic subjects showed that after a number of tasks were given in hypnosis, half completed and half interrupted, the subjects preferred the completed tasks both in the hypnotic state and in the "normal" state which followed directly. In order to investigate this finding, an hypothesis was set up according to which the subject regarded the interruption as a prohibition (because of the strong affective relationship between the experimenter and the hypnotic subject); and as a result of this, the interrupted tasks, it was supposed, were "avoided" by the subject.

In an attempt to check this hypothesis, control experiments were carried out with two groups of college students in the normal state. In one group, the interruption was "prohibitive"; in the other, it was "mild". The "prohibitive group" like the hypnotic subjects, preferred (and recalled) *relatively* more completed tasks than did the "mild group".[33] Apparently, then, when the field conditions are so varied as to set into operation a need that is more "central" than the "quasi-need" to complete an interrupted task, the "Zeigarnik effect" is accordingly modified. That this "central" need can be a powerful one in hypnosis is indicated by the fact that a mild interruption during hypnosis had results roughly equivalent to a severe prohibition in the normal state with the control subjects.

It may be tentatively concluded, thus, that a "tension system" created in hypnosis may have observable influence on behavior in the normal state, even though the subject has no awareness of the existence of such a "tension system" nor of its origins. The precise character of this influence is apparently related to the more "central needs" created either by the hypnotic relationship itself or by specific instructions during the course of the experiment.

[33] This finding requires support from further experiments with additional control subjects in order to attain statistical reliability. However, the trend in this direction is unmistakable.

(2) Attempts to Discharge a "Tension System" Created in Hypnosis by Task-Completion in Normal State

Statement of the Problem: The second problem investigated was whether a "tension system" created in the hypnotic state could be "discharged" by the completion in the "normal" state of those tasks that had been interrupted in the hypnotic state.[34]

Procedure with Alice A.: It will be recalled that the first half of the experiment with Alice A. was concerned with the problem of the influence on the normal state of a "tension system" created in the hypnotic state. The experimental account brought Alice A. to the point where she was brought out of hypnosis with amnesia for the Zeigarnik experiment and in this normal state preferred seven *completed* tasks and only three interrupted tasks in the ten pairs. It is at this juncture that the investigation of the second problem, that of the "discharge" of the "tension system", begins.

In the normal state, thus, Alice A. was permitted to complete the tasks originally interrupted in hypnosis, was then returned to the hypnotic state with amnesia for this completion, and asked for both recall and task preference. (Her amnesia was partially resolved by the experimenter who told her that she had "been doing some tasks" and that "some of them will come back to you now".)

Results with Alice A.: In striking contrast to her previous attitude in the "normal" state prior to completing the interrupted tasks, she now in the hypnotic state gave clear evidence for an *undischarged* "tension system" related to a "quasi-need"

---

[34] In the Zeigarnik (51) and Ovsiankina (34) experiments, it had been shown that after the interrupted tasks were completed, there was apparently no longer a "quasi-need" to do the interrupted tasks, thus indicating that the "tension system" had been "discharged". This problem was conceived prior to any actual experimentation, and was based on the premise that the Zeigarnik experiment conducted in hypnosis would result in a recall or preference advantage for the interrupted tasks. Despite the fact that the results of the experiments with Alice A. and with Barbara B. indicated a preference for the completed tasks both in hypnosis and in the following normal state after the Zeigarnik experiment, the experiment was carried out according to plan directly following the procedures discussed in the previous accounts of Alice A. and Barbara B.

to complete the interrupted tasks. She recalled[35] four interrupted tasks and only one completed task, yielding a Zeigarnik quotient of 4.0. Also, in contrast with her previous preferences of only three interrupted and seven completed tasks, she now preferred six interrupted and four completed tasks, yielding a "preference-quotient" of 1.5 as compared with a previous one of .42. Before discussing these results, a description will be given of a repetition of this experiment with Barbara B.

Procedure and Results with Barbara B.: Exactly the same procedure was followed in this experiment with similar results. After completing the tasks in the normal state Barbara was returned to the hypnotic state and asked for recall and preferences. She recalled six interrupted and three completed tasks, yielding a quotient of 2.0. Her preference-quotient "rose" from .42 (three interrupted and seven completed tasks) to 1.5 (six interrupted and four completed). Upon being returned once again to the normal state, with the posthypnotic suggestion that she would be able to recall some of the tasks, she recalled six interrupted and four completed tasks, a quotient of 1.5.

Discussion. Apparently something of vital dynamic significance had occurred between the time both subjects were asked for task-preferences in the normal state directly following the experiment in hypnosis, and the second hypnotic state. Behaviorally, the task-completion was the important intervening experience. However, in the usual Zeigarnik experiment, completion of the interrupted tasks should discharge the "tension system". In these two experiments, the attempted resolution in the normal state of a "tension system" originated in the hypnotic state had a diametrically opposite effect: it brought to the surface the strong "quasi-need" for completion of the tasks. If this result is tentatively interpreted along the same lines as the previous finding, then one might say that this sudden flaring up of the need to complete the interrupted tasks gives further evidence that this experimental situation

---

[35] This recall goes up to the first long pause which characteristically occurs after a few tasks have been recalled in rapid succession.

had induced two needs, one more "central" than the other, and that when the pressure of one was relaxed, the other could then be expressed. The "permission" to complete the tasks in the normal state apparently had the effect not of discharging the "tension system" but only of removing the "prohibition".

(3) Discharge of a "Tension System" Created in Hypnosis by Task-Completion in the Hypnotic State

Statement of the Problem: It had been predicted that although a "tension system" created in hypnosis[36] could not be discharged by task-completion in the normal state, it probably could be discharged by task-completion in a subsequent hypnotic state. Accordingly, a new experimental situation was set up to check on the latter half of this prediction.

Procedure: The procedure was described earlier[37] up to the point where Alice A. had been given the Zeigarnik experiment in the hypnotic state and had indicated her preference for the completed tasks in the normal state directly following. It was, thus, essentially a repetition of the other two experiments except for the fact that nonsense syllables were used. However, an additional step was taken to test the above hypothesis. This was not described in the earlier account because it is, logically, an independent problem.

Task completion in the normal state was permitted, with results similar to those just described: completion in the normal state had absolutely no effect on preference in the normal state[38] and when Alice A. was returned to hypnosis, she re-

[36] It should be emphasized that although it appeared that a "tension system" in Zeigarnik's sense was not created in the first hypnotic state, there can be little question that a real disequilibrium was produced as evidenced by the preference-shifts in the direction of the completed tasks. We infer thus that the need to complete the unfinished task was imbedded in the deeper wish to "please" or "obey" the experimenter.

[37] See p. 228.

[38] When returned from hypnosis to the normal state, having just done the Zeigarnik experiment, she preferred four interrupted and six completed tasks (quotient of .66). These figures were the same after completion in the normal state.

called (after her amnesia was partially resolved) seven interrupted and five completed tasks, yielding a quotient of 1.4.
Her preference-quotient, however, remained unchanged (.66).

It was at this point that the critical additional step was
taken: still in hypnosis, Alice A. *again* completed the interrupted tasks and was asked immediately in hypnosis for her
preferences. Apparently, this questioning was too soon on the
heels of the task-completion as no change had yet taken
place. However, when she was brought back to the normal
state and asked for task-preferences, Alice A. preferred five
interrupted and five completed tasks, yielding a quotient of
1.0 which, of course, is what would be obtained where no
"quasi-need" was present either to do the interrupted or the
completed tasks, i.e., a system in equilibrium.

Discussion: The results of this last experiment suggest that
the "discharge" of a tension system created in hypnosis can be
expected only in hypnosis; it appears that physical task-completion in the normal state does not "discharge" the tension
system and that it is necessary for this completion to take
place in hypnosis in order to restore an equilibrium in which
neither interrupted nor completed tasks are favored.

(4) The Revival of a "Tension System" by an Hypnotic "Regression"[39].

Statement of the Problem. This experiment was set up with
two fundamental objectives: (1) to see whether a technique
of hypnotic "regression" could be applied to so transitory an
experience as the "quasi-need" to complete interrupted tasks
and (2) to observe the nature of the "regressed quasi-need"
and its relation to the originally observed structure of the
"tension system" created in hypnosis.

Procedure: Three months after the first experiment with
Alice A.[40] she was experimentally "regressed" to the specific

---

[39] The term "regression" here refers to a re-orientation in hypnosis to an earlier
time. It is not used either in a Freudian or a Lewinian sense.

[40] See p. 224.

day on which the experiment proper had taken place. Alice A. was first told while in deep hypnosis that she had forgotten first the day, then the month, and finally the year. After this initial period of temporal disorientation she was re-oriented to the day of the experiment and told that she would no longer have any feeling of doubt regarding the date, month, and year but would be certain it was the day of the experiment. At this point, Alice A. began to perspire and complain of the heat and stuffiness of the room. Inasmuch as the "regression" experiment took place on a day in mid-winter, these reactions were somewhat puzzling until it was recalled that the day on which the original experiment had taken place had been one of the hottest of the Kansas summer. When it seemed established that this re-orientation was accepted by Alice A., she was told that she had just been doing some tasks and that she would recall some of them now.

Results: Alice A.'s recall, taken up to the first long pause, showed a 400 per cent advantage in memory for the interrupted tasks: she recalled five interrupted tasks and one completed.[41] (Zeigarnik quotient equals 5.0.) Her manner showed a great deal of tension and she seemed disturbed.[42] She enumerated also two tasks which she had seen several days prior to the experiment proper during a preliminary training period. This would indicate that the experimental "regression" was not so thorough-going that it entirely abrogated all standard "memory-laws". Yet it must be emphasized that "regression"-

---

[41] She recalled these tasks from the experiment in the following order:

Interrupted: 1. Cut out sport outfit. *Completed:* 6. Block design.
2. Ground plan.
3. Jig-saw puzzle.
4. Cross-word puzzle.
5. Mathematical problems.

[42] It seems likely from this and other studies of hypnotic "regression" that the process of re-orientation puts a severe strain on the subject and that unless the subject has an extended period of training for such "regression", it is difficult for him to remain "regressed" for long periods.

to a specific day after a lapse of three months requires an extremely delicate discrimination.

Discussion: In Zeigarnik's original experiment the average advantage in memory for the interrupted tasks directly following the experiment was 90 per cent. Also, an advantage of 110 per cent dropped within twenty-four hours to only 13 per cent. In the above report, the 400 per cent advantage of the interrupted tasks appears therefore especially striking. This result suggests that the re-activation of the "quasi-need" to complete the interrupted tasks took place in a highly charged setting dominated by a strong wish to please the experimenter. If there had been no need induced to complete the tasks, the subject would likely have shown only the usual hypnotic hypermnesia, and would have recalled a greater number of both interrupted and completed tasks than if the experiment had been conducted in the normal state. It seems likely that the essential factor in this result is the intensity of the hypnotic relationship which served to reinforce the re-activated "tension system", i.e., the original task-interruption determined *which* tasks would be recalled; the hypnosis determined how many. In order to further extend this hypothesis it would be necessary to do the same experiment with a hypnotic subject in the *normal* state and then effect a "regression" to the normal state after a similar period. This would indicate whether it was the "hypnotic regression" or the original creation of the "tension system" in hypnosis that produced the 400 per cent advantage in memory for the interrupted tasks.

(5) A Comparison of "Normal" and Hypnotic Zeigarnik Quotients

Statement of the Problem: The hypothesis regarding the preference for completed tasks[43] after the Zeigarnik experiment in hypnosis was based on three experiments. It was felt that perhaps in these three cases, the personalities of the subjects might have determined a low quotient, with or with-

[43] See pp. 229-230.

out hypnosis. Therefore, it seemed necessary to establish the "normal quotients" of a good hypnotic subject and compare those directly with the "hypnotic quotients".[44]

Subject used: Carol C., aged twenty-three, is a young stenographer; she volunteered for the experiment and although she was not quite so good a subject as Alice A., developed a good "trance" during the first individual session. She had seen hypnosis once as part of a vaudeville show which she had attended at about the age of eight. Despite the fact that her friends wondered at her not being afraid of hypnosis, she continued to come to the laboratory.

Procedure. In the normal state, Carol C. was asked her preferences between ten pairs of tasks.[45] Then, still in the normal state, she was given the twenty tasks to do and allowed to complete only half. She was asked for recall and again for preferences. Directly following this, amnesia for the entire experiment was produced in hypnosis. Five days later, she was given the Zeigarnik experiment in hypnosis and again asked for recall and preferences (still in hypnosis).

Results. After the experiment in the *normal* state, Carol C.'s preferences had shifted in the direction of the completed tasks. Her original preferences *before* the experiment had been for four interrupted and six completed tasks (quotient, .66); this differs from the usual "preperformance quotient" of 1.0 because the division of U and C tasks was kept the same as in the experiment with Barbara B., but Carol's preperformance preferences differed from Barbara's. After it, her quotient "dropped" to .33.[46] Her recall in the normal state totalled seven unfinished and six completed tasks. (Quotient is 1.16, a 16 per cent "advantage" for the unfinished tasks.)

[44] It is a well-accepted view among investigators in hypnosis that the best "control" for a given hypnotic subject is the same subject in the normal state.

[45] These were the same as those used in the experiment with Barbara B. See p. 226.

[46] Preferences before and after experiment:
Before: 1, 4, 6, 8, 9, 12, 13, 16, 17, 20. After: 1, 4, 5, 8, 10, 12, 14, 16, 18, 20.
The tasks corresponding to these numbers have been listed on p. 226 (foot-

After the experiment in the hypnotic state, her recall totalled six interrupted and seven completed tasks (quotient is .85, a 15 per cent "disadvantage" for the interrupted tasks). Because of interfering circumstances, the "preference-quotient" could not be obtained in this experiment.

Discussion: This experiment seems one of the least clear-cut in this series and therefore permits of many possible interpretations. First, it would appear that the central problem had been settled by the fact that Carol C. favored the interrupted tasks in her normal recall and the completed tasks in her hypnotic recall. However, it will be noticed that both of these trends are only trends and not sharply opposed, quantitatively. The 16 per cent advantage of the unfinished tasks is far below the average advantage (90 per cent) reported by Zeigarnik. Although this low quotient may be determined by a number of "non-hypnotic" factors, it seems additionally probable that the interpersonal relation existing between the experimenter and a hypnotic subject influences behavior *to some extent* in the normal as well as in the hypnotic state. A future experiment is thus logically dictated in which the "normal" Zeigarnik experiment will be given the subject by a person who is completely divorced from the hypnotic situation.

Secondly, the recall quotient of .85 does not indicate a decided tendency to favor the completed tasks (ratio, 6/7). In order to check this further, an experiment might be set up similar to the previously described normal "controls"[47] during the course of which the quality of the interruption might be varied systematically, and its effect on the recall quotient observed.

Finally, a new experiment must be set up in which the hypnotic experiment *precedes* the normal one; this, again, would

[47] See p. 230.

---

note). In the "after" calculations tasks 8 and 10 were omitted because although originally designated as C-tasks they were given as U-tasks to supplant others too quickly finished and therefore did not occupy the same position as in the original listing. Of the 8 tasks considered in the calculation then, 2 had been interrupted and 6 completed, yielding an "after" preference-quotient of .33.

safeguard against the possibility of producing a low recall quotient which is a result of a repetition of the experiment[48] and not of the peculiar affective character of the hypnotic state.

If, when all of these factors have been systematically controlled, the results still indicate a lower recall quotient *in the same individual* in hypnosis, then the hypothesis of interference by a more central need will be nearer "proof".

(6) An Experiment on Hallucinated Task-Completion in Hypnosis

Statement of the Problem: It had been suggested by some investigators[49] that the recall of tasks performed might frequently be influenced by the type of reaction aroused by the specific conditions of the experiment: that, for example, an experience of failure might result in the forgetting of a specific interrupted task. Accordingly, it was the aim of this experiment to see whether one could manipulate the attitudes toward various tasks by the creation of subjective reactions entirely independent of the objective or physical performance of the tasks.

Procedure: This experiment started at that point in the previously described experiment with Carol C. when Carol had just been through the Zeigarnik experiment in hypnosis. She was now brought back to the normal state and asked for recall (she had completed only half of the tasks in hypnosis, of course). Her recall totalled eight interrupted and seven completed tasks, yielding a recall quotient of 1.11 (an 11 per cent advantage for the interrupted tasks). Now she was again deeply hypnotized and told to hallucinate all of the tasks, one by one, and to "actually" complete them all at this hallucinated level. After each task that had been interrupted in the previous hypnosis, she was told that she had done "very poorly" or "much below average" and after each that had been a completed task she was told that she had done it "very well" or "much above

[48] See Pachauri (35) on this point.
[49] See discussion of Rosenzweig (40).

average". Although her total time in "completing" these hallucinated tasks was slightly shorter than it had been when she
had actually performed the tasks, the proportionate times she
took for each was in striking agreement with her objective time
taken previously. She was asked for recall and task-preference
and amnesia was produced for this experiment. The same procedure was then repeated except that the "praise" and "blame"
were reversed: the interrupted tasks were now given approba-
tory comments and the completed tasks, disapproving comments.

Results: Carol C.'s recall quotient after the first part of this
experiment[50] dropped from 1.11 (in the previous "normal"
state) to 1.0. She recalled seven interrupted and seven completed tasks. Her task-preference showed a striking shift: in
contrast to her original task preferences in the normal state
before any of these experiments (quotient, .66), she now produced a quotient of .11 (i.e., she preferred *all* the *completed*
tasks but one, the mosaic design). Thus, her preference for
those tasks that had been "praised" was unmistakable. After
the second half, her preference quotient rose slightly (quotient, .25) and her recall quotient remained 1.0. Thus, in response to the "praise" of the unfinished tasks the differential
between the U and C tasks decreased.

Discussion: The most significant implication of this experiment is that it suggests the possibility of directly manipulating
a "quasi-need" by the experimental introduction of a stronger,
more central need.[51] It suggests, too, that the objective source
of such a need may lie simply in an affective relationship and
not in the "real" results of "real" behavior. Further, it opens
a new path for the study of substitution. Lewin (26) reports
a study by Mahler of "substitute activities of different degrees
of reality" in which Mahler found that substitute activities of

[50] In the first half, the unfinished tasks were "blamed" and the completed tasks
"praised". The reverse was done in the second half.

[51] This formulation would correspond roughly to Rosenzweig's distinction
between an "ego-defensive" and a "need-persistive" reaction. (Cf. p. 218.)

"higher degrees of reality have greater substitute value". Yet hallucinated task-completion apparently "discharged" the "tension system" in this experiment. This finding, if it is found to be valid, thus focuses attention on another aspect of Mahler's discussion of his experiment which Lewin (26) has summarized as follows:

> "The relation of the substitute act to the inner goal of the original activity nevertheless remains of decisive importance. Substitute satisfaction occurs only when this inner goal is in sufficient degree attained by the substitute activity."[52]

If the "inner goal" of a good hypnotic subject is to "obey" or to "please" the experimenter, it is thus not difficult to see why it is theoretically to be expected that hallucinated task-completions have results very similar to those of actual task-completions. This experiment serves only to raise the question; in order to answer it, a systematic series of experiments would have to be set up involving varying reality-levels in *both* hypnotic and normal states.

(7) Summary and Discussion

These experiments have been described as aspects of various relatively independent logical problems. Although it was indicated that frequently a single experiment included the investigation of several distinct problems, the precise temporal relationships of the sub-sections of the single experiments may have been ambiguous. For this reason, we have included Table IV which summarizes the individual *hypnotic* experiments.[53] The control experiments have been adequately summarized earlier.[54] These figures are thus longitudinal summaries of the experience of the individual subject, in contrast with the

[52] p. 249.

[53] Cf. pp. 251-2.

[54] Cf. p. 236.

cross-sectional summaries, verbally presented in the subdivisions (1) through (6).

It must be emphasized that inasmuch as the experiments have been exploratory, the conclusions must be considered as hypotheses subject to modification or even reversal in terms of the results of further experimentation. These experiments have tried to crystallize a number of uninvestigated problems and to suggest "provable" or "disprovable" hypotheses for those problems specifically investigated. It is with all of these qualifications that the following conclusions are offered: (1) It appears that a "tension system" created in hypnosis has an observable influence on behavior in the normal state although the subject is unaware of its origins. (2) The discharge of a "tension system" appears to be an irreversible process as between normal and hypnotic states, i.e., a "tension system" created in hypnosis can apparently not be discharged by task-completion in the normal state, but can be by task-completion in the hypnotic state. It should be stated, however, that there is as yet no indication that the reverse is also true: namely, that a "tension system" created in the normal state may not be discharged in hypnosis. The results of experiments designed to investigate this latter problem will possibly indicate the relative boundary "permeability" of both normal and hypnotic states, thus offering a clue on the basis of which the topology of hypnotic states may be established. (3) The intensity of a hypnotically re-activated "tension system" seems more marked than that "normally" created. This conclusion is based on the "regression" experiment. (4) A comparison of the normal and hypnotic recall-quotients in the same subject, the preference- and recall-quotients in three additional experiments, and the results of a control experiment suggest that the interruption in hypnosis may be regarded as a "prohibition" by the subject. When task-completion is permitted in the normal state it may be that the "taboo" is lifted for the hypnotic subject allowing the emergence of the "quasi-need" to complete the tasks. (5) The attractiveness of a task may be manipulated, within limits, in hypnosis by the experimental creation of subjective feelings of "success" or "failure" even in the absence of physical performance. This refers to the experiment in which the hallucinated task-performances took place.

Perhaps the most puzzling question raised by these experiments is the problem of what Lewin has recently called[55] "changes in valence", i.e., " . . . change in attractiveness of an activity A as a result of an increase in the need tension in activity B, as distinguished from 'substitute value', that is, the degree to which completing A satisfies the need for B." It will be noted that in the normal control experiments, thirteen out of sixteen subjects preferred the completed tasks after taking part in the Zeigarnik experiment. Of the three who did not, two preferred the U and the C tasks equally[56] and one preferred six interrupted and four completed tasks.[57] Although this preference for the completed tasks was expected in the "prohibitive" group, it was not expected in the "mild" group. The possibility that this preference for the C-tasks lay in the nature of the tasks themselves was made doubtful by the fact that an independent equivalent group of thirteen students judged both U and C tasks "preferable" equally often.[58]

Cartwright (11) has investigated this problem and suggests that at least two factors must be distinguished as determining the attractiveness of an interrupted activity: (1) the increase of "valence" as a result of the need tension after interruption and (2) the fact that interruption may mean psychological failure and completion, success. (This past success and failure, he feels, may increase or decrease the attractiveness of an activity.)

[55] Private communication.

[56] Cf. Table I, p. 232.

[57] Cf. Table II, p. 233.

[58] This group simply judged the tasks without actually doing them. In order to rule out this possibility entirely, an experiment should be set up in which *all* tasks are completed and then judged for "attractiveness".

Yet another possibility is suggested by the fact that, while the resumption may perhaps be understood in terms of fulfilling a social expectancy, a statement of preference (where the subject no longer remembers whether the task was a U or a C task) may not be so understood. An experiment is thus suggested in which the subject is reminded at the time of his preferences that he did not finish this task and that he did finish that one.

In any case, it is clear that there is no simple relationship between the established indices of a "quasi-need" (better recall of U tasks and resumption) and the phenomenon of "preference". It is indicated, as well, that the needs evoked by the method of interruption must be considered in *any* experiment dealing with the problem of the effects of interruption. An extension of Cartwright's investigation as well as the control experiments suggested will unquestionably help to clarify this problem.

Whether or not further investigation would substantiate the specific findings of these experiments or the hypotheses used to explain them seems to us of minor significance. It was not our original intention to establish indisputable "content" in these experiments but rather to illustrate a method of research, using hypnosis as a tool. We feel that the potentialities of hypnosis in the experimental creation of needs of various intensities and on different levels might well be exploited to study the complex stratification of such needs and their dynamic interplay.[59]

[59] Taylor (45), in a study of memory theory, has advanced a view which is tangential to our assumptions here. He distinguishes three groups of "functional relata" within the psychological field: (1) the "environmental relata" which define the relationship of the organism to the external environment; (2) the "intrapersonal relata" which represent the differentiation of the individual; (3) the "intrafigural relata" which are responsible for the *structure* of the memory experience. Thus, according to Taylor, in the Zeigarnik experiment the interrupted tasks were at a *disadvantge* in terms of intrafigural relations but ". . . set up tensions in the intrapersonal field which more than overcame the disadvantage of the uncompleted tasks . . ." (p. 67). Thus, an apparent contradiction between the theory of Koffka (which stresses intrafigural relata) and that of Lewin (which stresses intrapersonal relata) is resolved. Although this view is in some ways different from the approach to the present research, its relevance is obvious.

TABLE IV

Figure 1.—Experiment with Alice A., using Meaningful Tasks.

N. S. No. 1	H. S. No. 1	N. S. No. 2	H. S. No. 2	H. S. No. 3 (3 mo. later)
P's asked in 10 pairs of tasks	Amnesia for N. S. No. 1	P's asked: PQ = .42	Recall asked: RQ = 4.0	"Regression" RQ = 5.0
	Zeigarnik experiment	Task completion	Preference asked:	
	Amnesia for H. S. No. 1		PQ = 1.5	

Figure 2.—Experiment with Alice A., using Nonsense Syllables.

N. S. No. 1	H. S. No. 1	N. S. No. 2	H. S. No. 2	N.S. No. 3
P.Q. = 1.0 (theoretically)	Zeigarnik experiment	P's asked: PQ = .66	Recall asked: RQ = 1.4 P's asked: PQ = .66	P's asked: P.Q. = 1.0
	P's asked: PQ = .42	Task-completion PQ = .66	Task-Completion PQ = .66	

Figure 3.—Experiment with Barbara B.

N. S. No. 1	H. S. No. 1	N. S. No. 2	H.S. No. 2	H.S. No. 3
P's asked: PQ = .66	Amnesia for N.S. No. 1	P's asked: PQ = .42	Recall asked: RQ = 2.0 P's asked: PQ = 1.5	R's asked: RQ = 1.5
	Zeigarnik Experiment	Task-Completion		
	Amnesia for H.S. No. 1			

Figure 4.—Experiment with Carol C.

N. S. No. 1	H. S. No. 1 (5 days later)	N. S. No. 2	H. S. No. 2
P's asked: PQ = 1.0	Zeigarnik Experiment: RQ = .85	RQ = 1.11	1. Told to hallucinate and perform tasks: C-tasks "praised": U-tasks "blamed": RQ = 1.0 PQ = .11
Zeigarnik Experiment	Posthypnotic suggestion for recall.		
Recall asked: RQ = 1.16 P's asked: PQ = .33			2. Reverse of (1): RQ = 1.0 PQ = .25
Amnesia			

NS., Normal State; H.S., Hypnotic State; P, Preference; R, Recall; Q, Quotient; U, Unfinished (task); C, Completed (task).

TABLE V

Order of Task Presentation in Experiment with Alice A.

1. Copy design (PC)
2. Cut out sport outfit (PU)
3. Manikin profile (PC)
4. Cut out tulip (NPC)
5. Block design (PC)
6. Plan of hospital grounds (PU)
7. Construct figure with match-sticks (NPU)
8. Do simple arithmetic problems (NPU)
9. Cut out design (NPC)
10. Number puzzle (PC)
11. Arrange panels to make joke (NPU)
12. Jig Saw (NPU)
13. Put together proverbs (NPC)
14. Plan of school grounds (NPC)
15. Actor, city, etc. with same initial (NPU)
16. Complete series of squares (NPC)
17. Build sentences (PC)
18. Cross Word puzzle (PU)
19. Fill in ellipses (PU)
20. Fill in blanks in sentences (PU)

P —Preferred

NP—Non-preferred

U —Unfinished

C —Completed

TABLE VI

I. Order of Presentation of Nonsense Syllables in Hypnotic
State in Experiment with Alice A.:

1. woer (C)
2. jish (C)
3. glet (C)
4. crad (U)
5. lerm (U)
6. sark (C)
7. goje (U)
8. hool (U)
9. fape (C)
10. kise (C)
11. roif (U)
12. twic (U)
13. theg (U)
14. chuz (C)
15. deux (U)
16. bune (C)
17. newk (C)
18. whab (U)
19. dolz (C)
20. kref (U)

II. Syllables Preferred in Hypnotic State after Zeigarnik Experiment: meor, jush, sark, hool, fape, kise, thog, whab, glet, bune.

III. Syllables Chosen in Normal State Following: weor, jish, crad, lerm, hool, fape, kise, bune, whab, dolz.

BIBLIOGRAPHY TO: HYPNOTHERAPY: A SURVEY OF THE LITERATURE

CHAPTER ONE

1. Bernheim, H. *Suggestive Therapeutics.* Translated by C. A. Herter. New York: G. P. Putnam's Sons, 1895.
2. Braid, J. *Neurypnology; Or, The Rationale of Nervous Sleep, Considered in Relation With Animal Magnetism.* London: G. Redway, 1899.
3. Bramwell, M. *Hypnotism: Its History, Practice and Theory.* Philadelphia: J. B. Lippincott Co., 1928 (Revised Edition).
4. Breuer, J. and Freud, S. *Studies in Hysteria.* Translated by A. A. Brill. New York: Nervous and Mental Disease Publishing Company, 1936.
5. Charcot, J. M. Oeuvres Complètes. *Metallotherapie et Hypnotisme.* Tome IX, Paris: Bourneville et E. Brissaud, 1890.
6. Dejerine, J. and Gauchler, E. *Psychoneuroses and Psychotherapy.* Translated by S. E. Jelliffe. Philadelphia: J. B. Lippincott, 1913.
7. Dessoir, M. *Bibliography of Modern Hypnotism.* Berlin: C. Dunckner, 1888.
8. DuBois, P. *Psychoneuroses and Their Psychic Treatment.* Bern: Francke, 1905.
9. Ferenczi, S. *Sex in Psychoanalysis.* Translated by E. Jones, Boston: Richard G. Badger, 1916. (See Chapter II on Introjection and Transference, originally published in the *Jahrbuch der Psychoanalyse*, 1909.)
10. Freud, A. *The Ego and the Mechanisms of Defence.* London: Hogarth Press, 1937.
11. Freud, S. *Autobiography.* Translated by J. Strachey. New York: W. W. Norton & Co., 1935.
12. ——— *Basic Writings.* Translated by A. A. Brill. New York: Modern Library, 1938.
13. ——— *General Introduction to Psychoanalysis.* Translated by G. S. Hall. New York: Horace Liveright, 1920.
14. ——— *Group Psychology and the Analysis of the Ego.* Translated by J. Strachey. London: The International Psychoanalytical Press, 1922.
15. ——— *History of the Psychoanalytic Movement.* Translated by A. A. Brill. New York: Nervous and Mental Disease Publishing Company, 1917.
16. Gurney, E. Recent Experiments in Hypnotism. *Proceedings of the Society for Psychical Research,* 5: 3, 1888.
17. Hart, B. *Psychopathology, Its Development and Its Place in Medicine.* New York: Macmillan Co., 1927.
18. Janet, P. *The Major Symptoms of Hysteria.* New York: Macmillan Co., 1907.
19. ——— *The Mental State of Hystericals.* New York: G. P. Putnam's Sons, 1901.
20. ——— *Principles of Psychotherapy.* Translated by H. M. and E. R. Guthrie. New York: Macmillan Co., 1924.
21. ——— *Psychological Healing, A Historical and Clinical Study.* Translated by E. and C. Paul. New York: Macmillan Co., 1925, 2 volumes.
22. Kiernan, J. G. Hypnotism in American Psychiatry Fifty Years Ago. *American Journal of Insanity,* 51: 336-354, 1894-95.
23. Liebault, A. *Du sommeil et des états analogues considérés surtout au point de vue de l'action morale sur le physique.* Nancy and Paris, 1866. Also, Vienna: F. Deuticke, 1892.

24. McDougall, W. Four Cases of "Regression" in Soldiers. *Journal of Abnormal Psychology*, 15: 136-156, 1920.
25. —— Hypnotism. *Encyclopaedia Britannica*, Eleventh Edition.
26. —— *Outline of Abnormal Psychology*. New York: Chas. Scribner's Sons, 1926.
27. Miller, H. C. *Hypnotism and Disease*. Boston: The Gorham Press, 1912.
28. Moll, A. *Hypnotism*. New York: Chas. Scribner's Sons, 1890.
29. Prince, M. *The Unconscious*. New York: Macmillan Co., 1914.
30. —— et al. *Psychotherapeutics*. Boston: The Gorham Press, 1912.
31. —— and Putnam, J. J. A Clinical Study of a Case of Phobia. *Journal of Abnormal Psychology*, 7: 259-292, 1912.
32. Schilder, P. and Kauders, O. *Hypnosis*. Translated by S. Rothenberg. Nervous and Mental Disease Monograph Series, No. 46, 1927.
33. Sidis, B. *Foundations of Normal and Abnormal Psychology*. Boston: Richard G. Badger, 1914.
34. —— *The Psychology of Suggestion*. New York: D. Appleton-Century Co., 1898.
35. —— *Psychopathological Researches*. New York: G. E. Stechert, 1902.
36. —— *Nervous Ills: Their Cause and Cure*. Boston: Richard G. Badger, 1922.
37. Zilboorg, G. *History of Medical Psychology*. New York: W. W. Norton & Co., 1941.

CHAPTER TWO

38. Baudouin, C. *Suggestion and Autosuggestion*. Translated by E. and C. Paul. New York: Dodd, Mead & Co., 1922.
39. Bechterew, W. V. What is Hypnosis? *Journal of Abnormal Psychology*, 1: 18-25, April 1906.
40. Bernheim, H. *Suggestive Therapeutics*. Translated by C. A. Herter. New York: G. P. Putnam's Sons, 1895.
41. Bramwell, M. *Hypnotism: Its History, Practice and Theory*. Philadelphia: J. B. Lippincott Co., 1928 (Revised Edition).
42. Brotteaux, P. *Hypnotisme et Scopochloralose*. Paris: Vigot Frères, 1936.
43. —— *L'hypnotisme Moderne*. Paris: Vigot Frères, 1938.
44. Coué, E. *Self-Mastery Through Conscious Autosuggestion*. New York: American Library Service, 1922.
45. Davis, L. W. and Husband, R. W. A Study of Hypnotic Susceptibility in Relation to Personality Traits. *Journal of Abnormal and Social Psychology*, 26: 175-182, 1931.
46. Coriat, I. H. The Experimental Synthesis of the Dissociated Memories in Alcoholic Amnesia. *Journal of Abnormal Psychology*, 1: 109-22, 1906.
47. Donley, J. The Clinical Use of Hypnoidization. *Journal of Abnormal Psychology*, August-September, 1908.
48. Erickson, M. H. The Applications of Hypnosis to Psychiatry. *Medical Record*, 150: 60-65, 1939.
49. Fisher, C. Hypnosis in Treatment of Neuroses Due to War and to Other Causes. *War Medciine*, 4: 565-576, December 1943.
50. Forel, A. *Der Hypnotismus oder die Suggestion und die Psycho-therapie; ihre psychologische, psychophysiologische und medizinische Bedeutung mit Einschluss der Psychoanalyse, sowie der Telepathiefrage; ein Lehrbuch für Studierende sowie für weitere Kreise*. 10. und 11. Aufl. Stuttgart: F. Enke, 1921.

51. Friedlander, J. W. and Sarbin, T. R. The Depth of Hypnosis. *Journal of Abnormal and Social Psychology*, 33: 453-475, 1938.
52. Grinker, R. R. Conference on Narcosis, Hypnosis, and War Neuroses. New York: Sponsored by the Josiah Macy, Jr. Foundation, January 1944, (Privately distributed).
53. —— and Spiegel, J. P. *War Neuroses in North Africa. The Tunisian Campaign (January-May 1943).* New York: Josiah Macy, Jr. Foundation, 1943.
54. Hadfield, J. A. War Neurosis: A Year in a Neuropathic Hospital. *British Medical Journal*, 1: 320, March 7, 1942.
55. —— Chapter on "Treatment by Suggestion and Hypnoanalysis," pp. 128-149 in *The Neuroses in War*, edited by Emanuel Miller. New York: Macmillan Co., 1940.
56. Horsley, J. S. *Narcoanalysis*. London: Oxford University Press, 1943.
57. Hull, C. L. *Hypnosis and Suggestibility*. New York: D. Appleton-Century, 1933.
58. Janet, P. *Principles of Psychotherapy*. Translated by H. M. and E. R. Guthrie. New York: Macmillan Co., 1924.
59. —— *Psychological Healing, A Historical and Clinical Study,* Cf. No. 21.
60. Kraines, S. H. *The Therapy of the Neuroses and Psychoses*. Philadelphia: Lea and Febiger, 1941.
61. Kubie, L. S. Manual of Emergency Treatment for Acute War Neuroses. *War Medicine*, 4, 6: 582-598, December 1943.
62. —— Use of Induced Hypnagogic Reveries in the Recovery of Repressed Amnesic Data. *Bulletin of the Menninger Clinic*, 7, 5-6: 172-82, September-November, 1943.
63. —— and Margolin, S. A Physiological Method for the Induction of States of Partial Sleep, and Securing Free Association and Early Memories in Such States. *Transactions American Neurological Association*, 1942.
64. —— The Process of Hypnotism and the Nature of the Hypnotic State. *American Journal of Psychiatry*, 100: 611-622, March, 1944.
65. Maclay, W. S. and Stokes, A. B. *Second Report on the Work and Organization of an Emergency Medical Service Neurosis Centre*. Mill Hill Emergency Hospital, January 1, 1941 to December 31, 1942. London: Warden & Company.
66. McDougall, W. *Outline of Abnormal Psychology*. New York: Chas. Scribner's Sons, 1926.
67. Moll, A. *Hypnotism*. New York: Chas. Scribner's Sons, 1890.
68. Neustetter, W. L. *Early Treatment of Nervous and Mental Disorders*. London: Churchill, 1940. (See chapter on The Technique of Hypnotism.)
69. Rogerson, C. H. Narcoanalysis with Nitrous Oxide. *British Medical Journal*, 1: 811-812, June 17, 1944.
70. Salter, A. Three Techniques of Autohypnosis. *Journal of General Psychology*, 24: 423-438, 1941.
71. —— *What Is Hypnosis?* New York: Richard R. Smith, 1944.
72. Sargent, W. and Fraser, R. Inducing Light Hypnosis by Hyperventilation. Lancet, 235: 778, 1938.
73. Schilder, P. and Kauders, O. *Hypnosis*. Nervous and Mental Disease Monograph Series, No. 46, 1927.
74. Sidis, B. *An Experimental Study of Sleep*. Boston: Richard G. Badger, 1909.

75. —— *Nervous Ills: Their Cause and Cure.* Boston: Richard G. Badger, 1922.
76. —— The Value of the Method of Hypnoidization in the Diagnosis and Treatment of Psychopathic Disorders. *Medical Times of New York,* xlvii, 245-250, 1919.
77. Stungo, E. Evipan Hypnosis in Psychiatric Outpatients. *Lancet,* April 19, 1941.
78. Vogt, O. Zur Kenntnis des Wesens und der psychologischen Bedeutung des Hypnotismus. *Zeitschrift fuer Hypnotismus,* 3: 277, 1894-95; 4: 32, 122, 229, 1896.
79. Wells, W. R. Experiments in Waking Hypnosis for Instructional Purposes. *Journal of Abnormal and Social Psychology,* 18: 389-404, 1924.
80. Wetterstrand, O. G. *Hypnotism and Its Application to Practical Medicine.* Translated by H. G. Petersen. New York: G. P. Putnam's Sons, 1902.
81. White, R. W. and Shevach, B. J. Hypnosis and the Concept of Disassociation. *Journal of Abnormal and Social Psychology,* 37: 3, 309-328, July 1942.
82. Wingfield, H. E. *An Introduction to the Study of Hypnotism, Experimental and Therapeutic.* London: Bailliere, Tindall & Cox, 1920.
83. Winkel, L. *Wesen and Bedeutung der therapeutischen Hypnose speciell bei Psychosen.* Bonn, P. Kubens, 1930.
84. Young, P. C. Is Rapport an Essential Characteristic of Hypnosis? *Journal of Abnormal and Social Psychology,* 22: 130-139, 1927.

CHAPTER THREE

85. Barry, H. Jr., MacKinnon, D. W. and Murray, H. A. Jr. Studies in Personality. A Hypnotizability as a Personality Trait and its Typological Relations. *Human Biology,* 3: 1-36, 1931.
86. Bartlett, M. R. Relation of Suggestibility to Other Personality Traits. *Journal of General Psychology,* 15: 191-196, 1936.
87. —— Suggestibility in Psychopathic Individuals: A Study with Psychoneurotic and Dementia Praecox Subjects. *Journal of General Psychology,* 14: 241-247, 1936.
88. Bernheim, H. *Suggestive Therapeutics.* Translated by C. A. Herter. New York: G. P. Putnam's Sons, 1895.
89. Bramwell, M. *Hypnotism: Its History, Practice and Theory.* Revised Edition. Philadelphia: J. B. Lippincott Co., 1928.
90. Brenman, M. and Reichard, S. Use of the Rorschach Test in the Prediction of Hypnotizability. *Bulletin of the Menninger Clinic,* 7: 5-6 183-187, 1943.
91. Copeland, C. L. and Kitching, E. H. Hypnosis in Mental Hospital Practice. *Journal of Mental Science,* 83: 316-329, 1937.
92. Davis, L. W. and Husband, R. W. A Study of Hypnotic Susceptibility in Relation to Personality Traits. *Journal of Abnormal and Social Psychology,* 26: 175-182, 1931.
93. Erickson, M. H. The Applications of Hypnosis to Psychiatry. *Medical Record,* 60-65, July 19, 1939.
94. Fisher, C. Hypnosis in Treatment of Neuroses Due to War and to Other Causes. *War Medicine,* 4: 565-76, December 1943.
95. Flatau, G. Experimenteller Hypnotismus. Vienna, *Psychotherapeut. Praxis,* 1: 155-159, 1934.

96. Forel, A. *Der Hypnotismus oder die Suggestion und die Psychotherapie; ihre psychologische, psychophysiologische and medizinische Bedeutung mit Einschluss der Psychoanalyse, sowie der Telepathiefrage; ein Lehrbuch für Studierende sowie für weitere Kreise*, 10. und 11. Aufl. Stuttgart: F. Enke, 1921.

97. Hull, C. L. *Hypnosis and Suggestibility*. New York: D. Appleton-Century, 1933.

98. Jenness, A. Chapter on Hypnotism. (In *Personality and the Behavior Disorders*, edited by J. McV. Hunt. New York: The Ronald Press, 1944, 2 volumes, pp. 466-502.)

99. ———— and Dahms, H. Change of Auditory Threshold during Reverie as Related to Hypnotizability. *Journal of General Psychology*, 17: 167-170, 1937.

100. Miller, H. C. *Functional Nerve Disease: An Epitome of War Experience for the Practitioner*. London: Oxford University Press, 1920.

101. Moll, A. *Hypnotism*. New York: Chas. Scribner's Sons, 1890.

102. Morgan, J. J. B. The Nature of Suggestibility. *Psychological Review* 31: 6, 1924.

103. Murray, H. *Explorations in Personality*. New York: Oxford University Press, 1938.

104. Rosenzweig, S. The Experimental Study of Repression. Pp. 472-91 in Murray's *Explorations in Personality*. New York: Oxford University Press, 1938.

105. ———— and Sarason, S. An Experimental Study of the Triadic Hypothesis: Reaction to Frustration, Ego-defense and Hypnotizability. *Character and Personality*, 11: 2, 1-19, December 1942.

106. Sarbin, T. R. and Madow, L. W. Predicting the Depth of Hypnosis by Means of the Rorschach Test. *American Journal of Orthopsychiatry*, 12: 2, 268-70, April 1942.

107. Schilder, P. Ueber das Hypnose-Erlebnis der Schizophrenie. *Zeitschrift für die gesamte Neurologie und Psychiatrie*, 120, 700-707, 1929.

108. Tuckey, C. L. *Treatment by Hypnotism and Suggestion or Psychotherapeutics*. London: Bailliere, Tindall & Co, 1921.

109. Vogt, O. Zur Kenntnis des Wesens und der psychologischen Bedeutung des Hypnotismus. *Zeitschrift fuer Hypnotismus*, 3: 277, 1894-95; 4: 32, 122, 229, 1896.

110. Voisin, J. Des réprésentations mentales et des hallucinations visuelles et auditives post-hypnotiques conscientes chez les personnes ayant subi le traitement hypnothérapeutique. *Cong. internat. de l'hypnot. expér. et therap.*, Paris, 276, 1902.

111. White M. M. The Physical and Mental Traits of Individuals Susceptible to Hypnosis. *Journal of Abnormal and Social Psychology*, 25: 293-98, 1930.

112. White, R. W. Hypnosis Test. Pp. 453-461 in Murray's *Explorations in Personality*, New York: Oxford University Press, 1938.

113. ———— Prediction of Hypnotic Susceptibility from a Knowledge of Subject's Attitudes. *Journal of Psychology*, 3: 265-277, 1937.

114. Williams, G. W. A Study of the Responses of Three Psychotic Groups to a Test of Suggestibility. *Journal of General Psychology*, 302-10, 1932.

115. Winkel, L. *Wesen und Bedeutung der therapeutischen Hypnose speciell bei Psychosen*. Bonn: P. Kubens, 1930.

CHAPTER FOUR

116. Bauer, C. Aus der hypnotischen Poliklinik des Herrn. Prof. Forel in Zürich, Sommersemester, 1896. *Zeitschrift für Hypnotismus*, Leipzig, Barth, 5: 31-45, 1897.

117. Bechterew, W. V. What is Hypnosis? *Journal of Abnormal Psychology*, 1: 18-25, April, 1906.

118. Beck, L. F. Hypnotic Identification of an Amnesia Victim. *British Journal of Medical Psychology*, 16: 36-42, 1938.

119. Bernheim, H. *Suggestive Therapeutics*. Translated by C. A. Herter. New York: G. P. Putnam's Sons, 1895.

120. Birnie, C. R. Anorexia Nervosa Treated by Hypnosis in Out-patient Practice. *Lancet*, 2: 1331-32, December 5, 1936.

121. Bonjour, J. La guérison des condylomes par la suggestion. *Schweizerische medizinische Wochenschrift*, 57: 980-81, 1927.

122. Bramwell, M. *Hypnotism: Its History, Practice and Theory*. Philadelphia: J. B. Lippincott Co., 1928.

123. Brenman, M. and Knight, R. P. Hypnotherapy for Mental Illness in the Aged: Case Report of Hysterical Psychosis in a 71-year-old Woman. *Bulletin of the Menninger Clinic*, 7: 5-6, 188-98, 1943.

124. —— Self-starvation and Compulsive Hopping with Paradoxical Reaction to Hypnosis. *American Journal of Orthopsychiatry*, 9: 65-75, 1945.

125. Breuer, J. and Freud S. *Studies in Hysteria*. Transl. by A. A. Brill, Nervous and Mental Disease Monograph Series, 1936.

126. Brickner, R. M. and Kubie, L. S. A Miniature Psychotic Storm Produced by Super-ego Conflict over Simple Posthypnotic Suggestion. *Psychoanalytic Quarterly*, 5: 467-87, 1936.

127. Brown, H. *Advanced Suggestion*. New York: William Wood & Co., 1919

128. Brown, W. Hypnosis in Hysteria. Letter to the Editor of the *Lancet*. 15: 505, October 5, 1918.

129. —— Hypnosis, Suggestibility and Progressive Relaxation. *British Journal of Psychology*, 28: 396-411, 1938.

130. —— *Psychology and Psychotherapy*. London: Edward Arnold & Co., 1934.

131. —— The Treatment of Cases of Shell-shock in an Advanced Neurological Centre. *Lancet*, 197-200, August 7, 1918.

132. —— Myers, C. S. and McDougall, W. Symposium on the Revival of Emotional Memories and its Therapeutic Value. *British Journal of Medical Psychology*, 1: 26, October 1920.

133. Bunnemann, O. Ueber psychogenes Ekzem. *Die Medizinische Welt*, 8: 87-88, 1934.

134. Carlill, H. Hypnotism. *Lancet*, 1: 61-66, January 5, 1935.

135. Connellan, P. S. The Treatment of Repressed Memories by Hypnotism. *Bristol Medical-Chirurgical Journal*, 43: 209-216, 1926.

136. Connelly, E. Uses of Hypnosis in Psychotherapy. *New Orleans Medical and Surgical Journal*, 88: 627-32, 1936.

137. Copeland, C. L. and Kitching, E. H. Hypnosis in Mental Hospital Practice. *Journal of Mental Science*, 83: 316-29, 1937.

138. Delius, H. Erfolge der hypnotischen Suggestiv-Behandlung in der Praxis. Leipzig, *Zeitschrift für Hypnotismus*, 5: 219-238, 1897.

139. Donley, J. E. The Clinical Use of Hypnoidization in the Treatment of Some Functional Psychoses. *Journal of Abnormal Psychology*, 3: 148-160, 1908-09.

140. Eisenbud, J. A. Method for Investigating the Effect of Repression on the Somatic Expression of Emotion in Vegetative Functions: a Preliminary Report. *Psychosomatic Medicine*, 1: 3, July 1939.
141. Erickson, M. H. Development of Apparent Unconsciousness During Hypnotic Reliving of a Traumatic Experience. *Archives of Neurology and Psychiatry*, 38: 1282-1288, 1937.
142. ———— The Induction of Color Blindness by a Technique of Hypnotic Suggestion. *Journal of General Psychology*, 20: 61-89, 1939.
143. ———— The Investigation of a Specific Amnesia. *British Journal of Medical Psychology*, 13: 143-150, 1933.
144. ———— A Study of Clinical and Experimental Findings on Hypnotic Deafness. (I) *Journal of General Psychology*, 19: 127-150, 1938. (II) *Ibid*, 19: 151-167, 1938.
145. ———— and Hill, L. Unconscious Mental Activity in Hypnosis, Psychoanalytic Implications. *Psychoanalytic Quarterly*, 13: 60-78, January 1944.
146. ———— and Kubie, L. S. The Permanent Relief of an Obsessional Phobia by Means of Communications with an Unsuspected Dual Personality. *Psychoanalytic Quarterly*, 8: 471-509, October 1939.
147. ———— The Successful Treatment of a Case of Acute Hysterical Depression by a Return under Hypnosis to a Critical Phase of Childhood. *Psychoanalytic Quarterly*, 10: 583-609, October 1941.
148. ———— The Use of Automatic Drawing in the Interpretation and Relief of a State of Acute Obsessional Depression. *Psychoanalytic Quarterly*, 7: 443-466, 1938.
149. Estrin, J. Hypnosis as Supportive Symptomatic Treatment in Skin Diseases: Cases. *Urologic and Cutaneous Review*, 45: 337-38, May 1941.
150. Farber, L. H. and Fisher, C. An Experimental Approach to Dream Psychology through the Use of Hypnosis. *Psychoanalytic Quarterly*, 12: 202-216, 1943.
151. Fervers, C. Analyse in Hypnose. *Der Nervenarzt*, 11: 25-30, January 1938.
152. Fisher, C. Hypnosis in Treatment of Neuroses due to War and to Other Causes. *War Medicine*, 4: 565-76, December 1943.
153. Forel, A. *Der Hypnotismus oder die Suggestion und die Psychotherapie; ihre psychologische, psychophysiologische und medizinische Bedeutung mit Einschluss der Psychoanalyse, sowie der Telepathiefrage; ein Lehrbuch für Studierende sowie für weitere Kreise.* 10. und 11. Aufl. Stuttgart: F. Enke, 1921.
154. Freud, S. *Autobiography.* Translated by J. Strachey. New York: W. W. Norton & Co., 1935.
155. Gerrish, F. The Therapeutic Value of Hypnotic Suggestion. *Journal of Abnormal Psychology*, 4: 99, 1909.
156. Gill, M. M. and Brenman, M. Treatment of a Case of Anxiety Hysteria by an Hypnotic Technique Employing Psychoanalytic Principles. *Bulletin of the Menninger Clinic*, 7: 5-6, 163-71, 1943.
157. Goldwyn, J. "Hypnoidalization": its Psychotherapeutic Value. *Journal of Abnormal Psychology*, 24: 170-185, 1929.
158. Grinker, R. R. and Spiegel, J. P. *War Neuroses in North Africa. The Tunisian Campaign (January-May 1943).* New York: Josiah Macy, Jr. Foundation, 1943.
159. Hadfield, J. A. Chapter on "Treatment by Suggestion and Hypnoanalysis." (In *The Neuroses in War*, edited by Emanuel Miller, New York: Macmillan & Co., 1940.)

160. —— The Reliability of Infantile Memories. *British Journal of Medical Psychology*, 13: 87-111, 1928.
161. —— Chapter on Hypnotism. (In *Functional Nerve Disease: An Epitome of War Experience for the Practitioner*. Edited by H. C. Miller. London: Hodder & Stoughton, Ltd., 1920.)
162. —— War Neurosis; a Year in a Neuropathic Hospital. *British Medical Journal*, 1: 320, March 1942.
163. Hart, H. H. Hypnosis in Psychiatric Clinics. *Journal of Nervous and Mental Diseases*, 74: 598-609, 1931.
164. Heyer, G. *Hypnosis and Hypnotherapy*. London: C. W. Daniel Co., 1931.
165. Hilger, W. *Hypnosis and Suggestion. Their Nature, Action, Importance, and Position Amongst Therapeutic Agents*. Translated by R. W. Felkin. New York: Rebman Co., 1921.
166. Hollander, B. *Hypnotism and Suggestion in Daily Life, Education and Medical Practice*. New York: G. P. Putnam's Sons, 1910.
167. —— *Methods and Uses of Hypnosis and Self-Hypnosis*. London: George Allen & Unwin, Ltd., 1935.
168. Hurst, A. F. and Symns, J. L. M. The Rapid Cure of Hysterical Symptoms in Soldiers. *Lancet*, 2: 139-141, August 3, 1918.
169. Janet, P. *The Major Symptoms of Hysteria*. New York: Macmillan Co., 1907.
170. —— *The Mental State of Hystericals*. Translated by C. R. Corson. New York: G. P. Putnam's Sons, 1901.
171. —— *Principles of Psychotherapy*. Translated by H. M. and E. R. Guthrie. New York: Macmillan Co., 1924.
172. —— *Psychological Healing, A Historical and Clinical Study*. Translated by E. and C. Paul. New York: Macmillan Co., 1925, 2 volumes.
173. Jentsch, E. Hypnologisches und Hypnotherapeutisches. Berlin: *Monatsschrift für Psychiatrie und Neurologie*, 45: 228-244, 1919.
174. Kardiner, A. *The Traumatic Neuroses of War*. Psychosomatic Medicine Monograph III. Washington: National Research Council, 1941.
175. Karamischew, A. J. Hypnotherapie bei Ekzem, bei Psoriasis. *Dermatologische Wochenschrift*, 102: 260-263, February 29, 1936
176. Keller, D. H. A Psychoanalytic Cure of Hysteria. Springfield, Illinois: *Institution Quarterly*, 8: 78-82, 1917.
177. Kohnstamm, O. Ueber den Einfluss der Hypnose auf Menstruationsstoerungen. *Die Therapie der Gegenwart*, 48: 354-59, 1907.
178. Kraines, S. H. *The Therapy of the Neuroses and Psychoses*. Philadelphia: Lea and Febiger, 1941. pp. 227-233.
179. Kroger, W. S. and Freed, S. C. The Psychosomatic Treatment of Functional Dysmenorrhea by Hypnosis. *American Journal of Obstetrics and Gynecology*, 817-822, December 1943.
180. Kubie, L. S. Manual of Emergency Treatment for Acute War Neuroses. *War Medicine*, 6: 582-98, December 1943.
181. Levbarg, J. J. Hypnosis: a Potent Therapy in Medicine. *New York Physician*, 14: 18, 1940.
182. Levine, M. *Psychotherapy in Medical Practice*. New York: Macmillan Co., 1942.
183. Lifschitz, S. Hypnoanalyse, *Abhandlungen aus dem Gebiete der Psychotherapie und medizinischen Psychologie*, 1930.
184. Lindner, R. M. *Rebel Without a Cause, The Hypnoanalysis of a Criminal Psychopath*. New York: Grune & Stratton, Inc., 1944.

185. Livingood, F. G. Hypnosis as an Aid to Adjustment. *Journal of Psychology,* 12: 203-7, 1941.
186. Loewenfeld, L. *Hypnotismus und Medizin.* Munich: J. F. Bergmann, 1922.
187. McDougall, W. Four Cases of Regression in Soldiers. *Journal of Abnormal Psychology,* 15: 136-156, 1920.
188. –––––– *Outline of Abnormal Psychology.* New York: Chas. Scribner's Sons, 1926.
189. –––––– The Revival of Emotional Memories and Its Therapeutic Value. *British Journal of Medical Psychology,* 1: 26, October 1920.
190. Milbrádt, W. and Kohler, A. Hypnoanalytic Therapy of Alleged Sciatica. *Die Medizinische Welt.* 8: 408, March 24, 1934.
191. Miller, E. *The Neuroses in War.* New York: Macmillan Co., 1940.
192. Miller, H. C. *Functional Nerve Disease.* London: Hodder and Stoughton, Ltd., 1920.
193. –––––– *Hypnotism and Disease.* Boston: The Gorham Press, 1912.
194. Moll, A. *Hypnotism.* New York: Chas. Scribner's Sons, 1890. Also Berlin, 1924.
195. Morgan, J. J. B. Hypnosis with Direct Psychoanalytic Statement and Suggestion in the Treatment of a Psychoneurotic of Low Intelligence. *Journal of Abnormal Psychology,* 19: 160-64, 1924.
196. Mott, F. W. *War Neuroses and Shell Shock.* New York: Oxford University Press, 1919.
197. Muhl, A. M. Automatic Writing Combined with Crystal Gazing as a Means of Recalling Forgotten Incidents. *Journal of Abnormal Psychology,* 19: 264-73, 1924.
198. –––––– Use of Automatic Writing in Determining Conflicts and Early Childhood Impressions. *Journal of Abnormal Psychology,* 18: 1-32, 1923.
199. Muniz, A. L. A Case of Anxiety Neurosis Cured by Hypnosis. *Revista medica cubana,* 47: 135-142, February 1936.
200. –––––– Hysteria, Mutism and Blindness Cured by Psychoanalysis and Hypnotism. *Revista medica cubana,* 48: 675-678, July 1937.
201. –––––– Hysterical Lethargy Cured by Hypnotism. *Revista medica cubana,* 46: 875-882, August 1935.
202. –––––– Incoercible Vomiting of Pregnancy Cured by Hypnosis. Havana: *Revista de la sanidad militar,* 6: 65-70, 1942.
203. Myers, C. S. The Revival of Emotional Memories and Its Therapeutic Value. *British Journal of Medical Psychology,* 1: 26, October 1920.
204. –––––– *Shell Shock* 1914-1918. Cambridge: University Press, 1940.
205. Neustatter, W. L. The Technique of Hypnotism. (In *Early Treatment of Nervous and Mental Disorders.* London: Churchill, 1940.)
206. Platonow, K. I. On the Objective Proof of the Experimental Personality Age Regression. *Journal of General Psychology,* 9: 190-209, 1933.
207. Prince, M. Automatic Writing Combined with Crystal Gazing. *Journal of Abnormal Psychology,* 20: 34, 1925-1926.
208. –––––– *The Dissociation of a Personality.* Second Edition. New York: Longmans, Green & Co., 1908.
209. –––––– *Clinical and Experimental Studies in Personality.* Second Edition. Edited by A. A. Roback. Cambridge: Sci-Arts, 1939.
210. –––––– and Coriat, I. Cases Illustrating the Educational Treatment of the Psycho-neuroses. *Journal of Abnormal Psychology,* 2: 166-177, 1907.
211. Renterghen, A. W. van. Ein Fall von Muskelkrampf (tic rotatoire). *Zeitschrift für Hypnotismus,* 4: 259-65, 1897.

212. Richter, P. *Das Stottern und seine Heilung durch hypnotische Suggestion.* Dresden: Rudolph, 1928.
213. Ross, T. A. *The Common Neuroses.* Baltimore: William Wood & Co., 1937.
214. ———— The Prevention of Relapse of Hysterical Manifestations. *Lancet,* 516-17, October 19, 1918.
215. ———— *Prognosis in the Neuroses.* Cambridge: University Press, 1936.
216. Rothenberg, S. Theories of Hypnosis and Its Use. *N. Y. State J. Med.* 28: 372-8, 1928.
217. Satow, L. *Hypnotism and Suggestion.* New York: Dodd, Mead & Co., 1923.
218. Schilder, P. *Psychotherapy.* New York: W. W. Norton & Co., 1938.
219. ———— and Kauders, O. *Hypnosis.* Translated by S. Rothenberg, Nervous and Mental Disease Monograph Series, No. 46, 1927.
220. Schulz, J. *Gesundheitsschaedigungen nach Hypnose.* Halle: C. Marhold, 1922.
221. Schwartz, O, *Psychotherapy and Psychogenesis of Corporeal Symptoms.* Vienna: Springer, 1925.
222. Scott, F. G. L. Ten Consecutive Cases Treated by Hypnotism. London: *Guy's Hospital Report,* 52: 114-119, 1913.
223. Sidis, B. *Nervous Ills, Their Cause and Cure.* Boston: Richard G. Badger, 1922.
224. ———— *Psychopathological Researches.* New York: G. E. Stechert, 1902.
225. Simmel, E. Private communication.
226. ———— *Psycho-analysis and the War Neuroses.* (Edited by Ernest Jones.) S. Ferenczi, K. Abraham, E. Simmel and E. Jones. London: International Psycho-analytical Press, 1921.
227. ———— War Neuroses. *Psychoanalysis Today.* New York: International University Press, 1944.
228. Smith, G. M. A Phobia Originating before the Age of Three—Cured with the Aid of Hypnotic Recall. *Character and Personality,* 5: 331-37, 1937.
229. Southard, E. E. *Shell-Shock and Other Neuropsychiatric Problems.* Boston: W. M. Leonard, 1919.
230. Speyer, N. and Stokvis, B. The Psychoanalytic Factor in Hypnosis. *British Journal of Medical Psychology,* 17: 217-222, 1938.
231. Stekel, W. *Psychoanalysis and Suggestion Therapy.* Translated by J. S. Van Teslaar. New York: Moffat Yard & Co., 1923.
232. Taplin, A. B. *Hypnotic Suggestion and Psycho-therapeutics.* London: Simpkin, Marshall, Hamilton, Kent & Co., Ltd., 1918.
233. ———— *Hypnotism and Treatment by Suggestion.* Liverpool: Littlebury Bros., 1928.
234. Taylor, W S. Behavior under Hypnoanalysis and the Mechanism of the Neurosis. *Journal of Abnormal Psychology,* 18: 107-124, 1923.
235. ———— A Hypnoanalytic Study of Two Cases of War Neurosis. *Journal of Abnormal Psychology,* 16: 344-55, 1921-22.
236. *Readings in Abnormal Psychology and Mental Hygiene.* New York: D. Appleton-Century, 1926.
237. ———— Three Cases Illustrating Mechanisms and Interpretations of Neuroses. (In: *Readings in Abnormal Psychology.*)
238. Tombleson, J. B. An Account of 20 Cases Treated by Hypnotic Suggestion. London: *Journal Royal Army Medical Corps,* 340-346, 1917.
239. Travis, R. C. A Study of the Effect of Hypnosis on a Case of Dissociation Precipitated by Migraine. *American Journal of Psychology,* 36: 207, 1925.

240. Trotter, R. H. Neurasthenic and Hysterical Cases in General Military Hospitals. *Lancet*, 703, November 23, 1918.
241. Tuckey, C. L. *Treatment by Hypnotism and Suggestion or Psychotherapeutics.* London: Bailliere, Tindall & Cox, 1921.
242. Wells, W. R. The Hypnotic Treatment of the Major Symptoms of Hysteria: a Case Study. *Journal of Psychology*, 17: 269-297, 1944.
243. Wetterstrand, O. G. *Hypnotism, and Its Application to Practical Medicine.* Translated by H. G. Petersen. New York: G. P. Putnam's Sons, 1902.
244. Winkel L. *Wesen und Bedeutung der therapeutischen Hypnose speciell bei Psychosen.* Bonn: P. Kubens, 1930.
245. Wisch, J. M. Anwendung der Hypnose bei Psoriasis. *Dermatologische Wochenschrift*, 100: 234-36, February 23, 1935.
246. Wittkower, E. Studies on the Influence of Emotions on the Functions of Organs. *Journal of Mental Science*, 81: 533, 1935.
247. Yealland, L. R. *Hysterical Disorders of Warfare.* New York: Macmillan & Co., 1918.
248. Yellowlees, H. *A Manual of Psychotherapy.* London: A. and C. Black, Ltd., 1923.
249. Young, P. C. Hypnotic Regression—Fact or Artifact? *Journal of Abnormal and Social Psychology*, 35: 273-278, 1940.
250. Zilboorg, G. *History of Medical Psychology.* New York: W. W. Norton Co., 1941.

CHAPTER FIVE

251. Alrutz, S. *Neue Strahlen des menschlichen Organismus,* (Kleine Schriften z. Seelenforsch. H. 9), Suttgart; Julius Puttmann, 1924.
252. Bass, M. J. Differentiation of the Hypnotic Trance from Normal Sleep. *Journal of Experimental Psychology*, 14: 382-99, 1931.
253. Bernheim, H. *Die Suggestion und ihre Heilwirkung.* Leipzig and Vienna: F. Deuticke, 1888.
254. Biermann, B. Der Hypnotismus im Lichte der Lehre von den bedingten Reflexen. *Journal für Psychologie und Neurologie*, 35: 265-81, 1929.
255. Braid, J. *Neurypnology: Or, The Rationale of Nervous Sleep, Considered in Relation with Animal Magnetism.* London: G. Redway, 1843.
256. Breuer, J. and Freud, S. *Studies in Hysteria.* Nervous and Mental Disease Monograph Series, 1936.
257. Brown, W. Hypnosis, Suggestion and Dissociation. *British Medical Journal*, June 14, 1919.
258. Cappie—cited by Stokvis. Cf. No. 286.
259. Charcot, J. M. *Poliklinische Vorträge.* Leipzig und Vienna: F. Deuticke, 2 volumes.
260. Coué, E. *Self Mastery Through Conscious Autosuggestion.* American Library Service, New York, 1922.
261. Davis, R. C. and Kantor, J. R. Skin Resistance during Hypnotic State. *Journal of General Psychology*, 13: 62-81, 1935.
262. Dollken—cited by Stokvis. Cf. No. 286.
263. Farber, L. H. and Fisher, C. An Experimental Approach to Dream Psychology through the Use of Hypnosis. *Psychoanalytic Quarterly*, 12, 2: 202-216, April 1943.
264. Ferenczi, S. Introjektion und Uebertragung. *Jahrbuch für Psychoanalyse und Psychopathologische Forschung*, 422-458, 1909.

265. Freud, S. *Group Psychology and the Analysis of the Ego.* Translated by J. Strachey. London: The International Psycho-analytical Press, 1922.
266. Grinker, R. R. and Spiegel, J. P. *War Neuroses in North Africa. The Tunisian Campaign (January-May 1943).* New York: Josiah Macy, Jr. Foundation, 1943.
267. Heidenhain, R. P. H. *Der sogenannte tierische Magnetismus.* Leipzig: Breitkopf & Hartel, 1890.
268. Heilig, H. and Hoff, H. Psychische Beeinflussung von Organfunktionen, insbesondere in der Hypnose. *Zeitschrift für Psychotherapie,* 268-280, 1928.
269. Hilger, W. *Die Hypnose und die Suggestion.* Jena: Gustav Fischer, 1925
270. Hull, C. L. *Hypnosis and Suggestibility.* New York: D. Appleton-Century, 1933.
271. Isserlin, M. *Psychotherapie.* Berlin: Julius Springer, 1926.
272. Janet, P. *The Major Symptoms of Hysteria.* New York: Macmillan Co., 1907.
273. Jenness, A. and Wible, C. L. Respiration and Heart Action in Sleep and Hypnosis. *Journal of General Psychology,* 16: 197-222, 1937.
274. Jones, E. The Nature of Auto-suggestion. *British Journal of Medical Psychology,* 3: 206-212, 1923.
275. Kubie, L. S. The Use of Induced Hypnagogic Reveries in the Recovery of Repressed Amnesic Data. *Bulletin of the Menninger Clinic,* 7: 5-6, 172-182 1943.
276. ———— and Margolin, S. The Process of Hypnotism and the Nature of the Hypnotic State. *American Journal of Psychiatry,* 100: 611-622, March, 1944.
277. Loomis, A. L., Harvey, E. N., and Hobart, G. Brain Potentials during Hypnosis. *Science,* 83: 239-241, 1936.
278. Lundholm, H. and Lowenbach, H. Hypnosis and the Alpha Activity of the Electroencephalogram. *Character and Personality,* 11, 2: 145-149, 1942.
279. McDougall, W. *Outline of Abnormal Psychology.* New York: Chas. Scribner's Sons, 1926.
280. Pavlov, I. P. Inhibition, Hypnosis and Sleep. *British Medical Journal,* 256-257, 1923.
281. Rado, S. The Economic Principle in Psycho-analytic Technique. *International Journal of Psycho-analysis,* 6: 35-44, 1935.
282. Rivers, W. H. R. *Instinct and the Unconscious.* Cambridge: University Press, 1922.
283. Salter, A. *What is Hypnosis?* New York: Richard R. Smith, 1944.
284. Schilder, P. and Kauders, O. *Hypnosis.* Translated by S. Rothenberg. Nervous and Mental Disease Monograph Series, No. 46, 118, 1927.
285. Sidis, B. *The Psychology of Suggestion.* New York: D. Appleton-Century, 1898.
286. Stokvis, B. B. *Byjdrage tot de kennis der psychologie en der hypnotherapie van essentieele hypertensie met behulp van de voortdurende, automatische bloeddrukregistreering.* N. V. uitgeversmaatschappij "de Tijdstroom," Lochem, 1937.
287. Trömner, E. *Hypnotismus und Suggestion,* Aus Natur und Geisteswelt No. 199, G. G. Teubner, Leipzig und Berlin, 1913.
288. Verworn, M. *Allgem. Physiologie.* Jena: Gustav Fischer, 1901.
289. Wells, W. R. Experiments in Waking Hypnosis for Instructional Purposes. *Journal of Abnormal and Social Psychology,* 18: 389-404, 1924.

290. White, R. W. A Preface to the Theory of Hypnotism. *Journal of Abnormal and Social Psychology*, 36: 477-505, October 1941.
291. ――― and Shevach, B. J. Hypnosis and the Concept of Dissociation. *Journal of Abnormal and Social Psychology*, 37: 3, 309-328, July 1942.
292. Young, P. C. A General Review of the Literature on Hypnotism. *Psychological Bulletin*, 24: 540-560, 1927.
293. ――― Suggestion as Indirection. *Journal of Abnormal and Social Psychology*, 26: 1, 69-90, April 1931.

CHAPTER SIX

294. Kubie, L. S. and Margolin, S. A Physiological Method for the Induction of States of Partial Sleep, and Securing Free Association and Early Memories in Such States. *Transactions American Neurological Association*, 1942.
295. Schilder, P. and Kauders, O. *Hypnosis*. Translated by S. Rothenberg. Nervous and Mental Disease Monograph Series, No. 46, 118, 1927.

BIBLIOGRAPHY TO: FOUR CASE STUDIES

1. Freud, Sigmund. *Interpretation of Dreams.* New York: Macmillan Co., 1933.
2. *Ibid.* Metapsychological Supplement to Theory of Dreams. *Collected Papers,* Vol. IV. London: Hogarth Press, 1924
3. Janet, Pierre. *Mental State of Hystericals.* New York: G. P. Putnam's Sons, 1901.
4. Gill, Merton M., and Brenman, Margaret. Treatment of a Case of Anxiety Hysteria by an Hypnotic Technique Employing Psychoanalytic Principles. *Bulletin of the Menninger Clinic,* 7: 5-6, 163-171, Sept.-Nov. 1943.
5. Kubie, L. S., and Margolin, S. The Process of Hypnotism and the Nature of the Hypnotic State. *American Journal of Psychiatry,* 100: 611-622, March 1944.
6. Alexander, George H. Anorexia Nervosa. *Rhode Island Med. J.,* 22: 1939.
7. Benedek, Therese. Dominant Ideas and Their Relation to Morbid Cravings. *International Journal of Psycho-analysis,* 17: 1, 1936.
8. Cross, Ernest S. The Diagnosis and Treatment of Anorexia Nervosa. *Medical Clinics of North America,* March 1939.
9. Eissler, K. R. Some Psychiatric Aspects of Anorexia Nervosa, Demonstrated by a Case Report. *Psychoanalytic Review,* 30: II, 1943.
10. Lorand, Sandor. Anorexia Nervosa, Its Psychodynamics and Treatment. *Psychosomatic Medicine,* 5: III, 1943.
11. Masserman, Jules H. Psychodynamisms in Anorexia Nervosa and Neurotic Vomiting. *Psychoanalytic Quarterly,* 10: 1941.
12. McCullagh, E. Perry, and Walter R. Tupper. Anorexia Nervosa. *Annals Internal Medicine,* 14: V, 1940.
13. Moulton, Ruth. A Psychosomatic Study of Anexoria Nervosa Including the Use of Vaginal Smears. *Psychosomatic Medicine,* 4: I, 1942.
14. Rahman, L., H. B. Richardson, and H. S. Ripley. Anorexia Nervosa. *Psychosomatic Medicine.* 1: 1939.
15. Richardson, H. B. Simmonds' Disease and Anorexia Nervosa. *Archives of Internal Medicine,* 63: 1, 1939.
16. Ryle, J. A. Anorexia Nervosa. *Lancet,* 2: 1936.
17. Waller, J. V., M. R. Kaufman and F. Deutsch. Anorexia Nervosa. *Psychosomatic Medicine,* 2: III, 1940.

BIBLIOGRAPHY TO: AN EXPERIMENTAL STUDY

1. Adler, D. L. The Experimental Production of Repression. *Proceedings of the Eighth Annual Meeting of Topological Psychologists*, 1940-41, pp. 27-36.
2. Adler, D. L. and Kounin, J. S. Some Factors Operating at the Moment of Resumption of Interrupted Tasks. *Journal of Psychology*, 7: 255-267, 1939.
3. Alexander, F. Psychoanalysis Revised. *Psychoanalytic Quarterly*, 9: 1-36, 1940.
4. Angyal, A. *Foundations for a Science of Personality*. The Commonwealth Fund. New York: Oxford University Press, 1941, 398 pages.
5. Barker, R., Dembo, T., and Lewin, K. Frustration and Regression, an Experiment with Young Children. Studies in Topological and Vector Psychology, II, *University of Iowa Studies*, Studies in Child Welfare, XVIII, 1, 1941.
6. Bernfeld, S. The Facts of Observation in Psychonanalysis. *Journal of Psychology*, 12: 289-305, 1941.
7. Brown, J. F. *The Psychodynamics of Abnormal Behavior*. New York: McGraw-Hill, 1940.
8. ————— Psychoanalysis, Topological Psychology and Experimental Psychopathology. *Psychoanalytic Quarterly*, 6: 227-237, 1937.
9. ————— The Position of Psychoanalysis in the Science of Psychology. *Journal of Abnormal and Social Psychology*, 35: 29-44, 1940.
10. ————— The Psychoanalytical and Topological Modes of Attack. *Proceedings of the Seventh Annual Meeting of Topological Psychologists*, 1939, pp. 1-7.
11. Cartwright, D. The Effect of Interruption, Completion and Failure Upon Attractiveness of Activities. (Unpublished paper.)
12. Diven, K. Certain Determinants in the Conditioning of Anxiety Reactions. *Journal of Psychology*, 3: 219-308, 1937.
13. Edwards, A. The Retention of Affective Experiences—a Criticism and Restatement of the Problem. *Psychological Review*, 49: 43-53, 1942.
14. Erickson, M. H. The Applications of Hypnosis to Psychiatry. *Medical Record*, 150: 60-65, 1939.
15. ————— Experimental Demonstration of the Psychopathology of Everyday Life. *Psychoanalytic Quarterly*, 8: 338-353, 1939
16. Fisher, R. A. *The Design of Experiments*. London: Oliver and Boyd, 1937.
17. Flanagan, D. The Influence of Emotional Inhibition on Learning and Recall. (Unpublished thesis on file, University of Chicago Library, 1930.)
18. Frank J. D. The Contributions of Topological and Vector Psychology to Psychology and Psychiatry. *Psychiatry*, 5: 15-22, 1942
19. French, T. M. Dreams as Means of Studying the Subjective Factors in Structuralization of the Field. *Proceedings of the Seventh Annual Meeting of Topological Psychologists*, 1939.
20. ————— Goal, Mechanism and Integrative Field. *Psychosomatic Medicine*, 3: 226-252, 1941.
21. Gould, R. An Experimental Investigation of Repression. *Proceedings of the Eighth Annual Meeting of Topological Psychologists*, 1940, pp. 39-61.
22. Horney, K. *New Ways in Psychoanalysis*. New York: W. W. Norton & Co., 1939.
23. Kardiner, A. Psychoanalysis and Psychology. *Philosophy of Science*, 6: 233-254, 1941.

270   HYPNOTHERAPY: A SURVEY OF THE LITERATURE

24. Katz, E. Some Factors Affecting Resumption of Interrupted Activities. University of Minnesota, Institute of Child Welfare.
25. Landis, C. Psychoanalysis and Scientific Method. *Proceedings of the American Philosophical Society*, 84: 4, 1941.
26. Lewin, K. *A Dynamic Theory of Personality*. New York and London: McGraw-Hill Book Co., 1935.
27. ———— *Principles of Topological Psychology*. New York: McGraw-Hill Book Co., 1936.
28. ———— Psychoanalysis and Topological Psychology. *Bulletin of the Menninger Clinic*, 1: 202-211, 1937.
29. ————, Lippitt, R., and Escalona, S. K. Studies in Topological and Vector Psychology. *University of Iowa Studies*, Studies in Child Welfare, Volume XVI, 3, 1940.
30. Luria, A. R. *The Nature of Human Conflicts*. New York: Liveright Publ. Corp., 1932.
31. MacKinnon, D. W. A Topological Analysis of Anxiety: an Attempt at a Rapprochement between Topological Psychology and Psychoanalysis. *Proceedings of the Seventh Annual Meeting of Topological Psychologists*, 1939, pp. 6-16.
32. Marrow, A. Goal Tensions and Recall. *Journal of General Psychology*, 19: 3-35, 1938.
33. Murray, H. A. *Explorations in Personality*. New York: Oxford University Press, 1939.
34. Ovsiankina, M. Untersuchungen zur Handlungs und Affektpsychologie; die Wiederaufnahme unterbrochener Handlungen. *Psychologische Forschung*, 11: 302-79, 1928. (Cf. Summary in Lewin's *A Dynamic Theory of Personality*, p. 242.)
35. Pachauri, A. R. A Study of Gestalt Problems in Completed and Interrupted Tasks. *British Journal of Psychology*, 25: 365-381, 447-457, 1935
36. Platonow, K. I. On the Objective Proof of the Experimental Personality Age Regression. *Journal of General Psychology*, 1: 190-209, 1933.
37. Pratt, C. *The Logic of Modern Psychology*. New York: Macmillan Co., 1939.
38. Rapaport, D. *Emotions and Memory*. Baltimore: The Williams & Wilkins Co., 1942.
39. ———— Freudian Mechanisms and Frustration Experiments. *Psychoanalytic Quarterly*, 9: 503-511, 1942.
40. Rosenzweig, S. Need-persistive and Ego-defensive Reactions to Frustration as Demonstrated by an Experiment on Repression. *Psychological Review*, 40: 4, 1941.
41. Schlote, W. Ueber die Bevorzugung unvollendeter Handlungen. *Zeitschrift für Psychologie*, 117: 1-72, 1930.
42. Sharp, A. A. An Experimental Test of Freud's Doctrine of the Relation of Hedonic Tone to Memory Revival. *Journal of Experimental Psychology*, 22: 395-418, 1938.
43. ———— The Influence of Certain Emotional Inhibitions on Learning and Recall. (Unpublished thesis on file, University of Chicago Library, 1930.)
44. Stalnaker, J. M. and Riddle, E. E. The Effect of Hypnosis on Long-delayed Recall. *Journal of General Psychology*, 6: 429-440, 1932.
45. Taylor, D. The Remembering of Visual Form: a Comparison of Theories of Memory. (Unpublished thesis on file, University of Kansas, 1940.)

46. Watson, K. B. *The Nature and Measurement of Musical Meanings.* Evanston, Ill.: American Psychological Association, 1942.
47. White, M. M. Evidence from Hypnosis of Inhibition as a Factor in Recall. (Abstract) *Psychological Bulletin,* 32: 689-690, 1935.
48. White, R. W., Fox, G. F., and Harris, W. W. Hypnotic Hypermnesia for Recently Learned Material. *Journal of Abnormal and Social Psychology,* 35: 88-103, 1940.
49. Wright, B. Altruism in Children and the Perceived Conduct of Others. *Journal of Abnormal and Social Psychology,* 37: 218-233, 1942.
50. Young, P. C. Experimental Hypnotism: a Review. *Psychological Bulletin,* 38: 92-104, 1941.
51. Zeigarnik, B. Das Behalten von erledigten und unerledigten Handlungen. *Psychologische Forschung,* 9: 1-85, 1927.

Certain recent publications in this field have not been included here, since the major portion of this study was concluded before 1942. A few of the significant additions to the literature are:

Masserman, J. *Behavior and Neurosis. An Experimental Psychoanalytic Approach to Psychobiologic Principles.* Chicago: University of Chicago Press, 1943.

Hunt, J. McV. *Personality and the Behavior Disorders.* New York: Ronald Press, 1944.

Sears, R. R. Survey of Objective Studies of Psychoanalytic Concepts. *Social Science Research Council Bulletin,* No. 51, New York, 1942.

Tomkins, S. S. *Contemporary Psychopathology.* Cambridge: Harvard University Press, 1943.

INDEX